Student Study Guide

to accompany

Fox's
Physiological Basis for
Exercise and Sport

Sixth Edition

Merle L. Foss
University of Michigan

Steven J. Keteyian
William Clay Ford Center for Athletic Medicine

Prepared by
Susan Muller
Salisbury State University

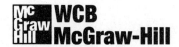

Boston   Burr Ridge, IL   Dubuque, IA   Madison, WI   New York   San Francisco   St. Louis
Bangkok   Bogotá   Caracas   Lisbon   London   Madrid
Mexico City   Milan   New Delhi   Seoul   Singapore   Sydney   Taipei   Toronto

WCB/McGraw-Hill

A Division of The McGraw·Hill Companies

Student Study Guide to accompany
FOX'S PHYSIOLOGICAL BASIS FOR EXERCISE AND SPORT, 6/E

2 3 4 5 6 7 8 9 0 CUS/CUS 9 0 9

ISBN 0-697-37618-4

www.mhhe.com

Table of Contents

CHAPTER 1
INTRODUCTION TO EXERCISE PHYSIOLOGY, SPORTS MEDICINE AND KINESIOLOGY

Lecture Preparation: Multiple Choice

Instructions: After reading the chapter, read each question and the answer choices. Select the choice which BEST answers the question. Check your answers at the back of this chapter, and review any incorrectly answered questions in your textbook.

Pretest

1. A calorimeter was first used to measure energy metabolism in
   a. cats
   b. dogs
   c. humans
   d. chimps

2. In 1847 von Helmholtz elucidated the law of
   a. thermodynamics
   b. conservation of momentum
   c. conservation of energy
   d. mass & acceleration

3. In 1913 Benedict & Cathcart published the classic study of the Human Body as
   a. machine
   b. compared to apes
   c. compared to dogs
   d. biomechanical devices

4. D.B. Dill served as the director of the Harvard
   a. school of science
   b. physical education department
   c. physiology department
   d. fatigue lab

5. The world's largest, most respected organization for sports and science
   a. ACE
   b. ACSM
   c. NATA
   d. NSCA

6. The _____ revolution was started in part by Dr. Kenneth Cooper
   a. physiology
   b. sports medicine
   c. fitness
   d. wellness

7. The US Surgeon General established this series of goals for the citizens of the USA
   a. healthy people 2,000
   b. presidential physical fitness test
   c. physical best test
   d. health Initiatives 2,000

8. In 1996, the Surgeon General reiterated the importance of
   a. not smoking
   b. getting enough sleep
   c. a balanced diet
   d. an active lifestyle

9. The USOC was established to
   a. get kids into sports
   b. coordinate the US Olympic efforts
   c. train our soldiers
   d. set national P.E. objectives

Key Terms - Define the following terms:

1. Exercise Physiology
2. Sports Medicine
3. Kinesiology
4. ACSM
5. NATA
6. AAHPERD
7. AWHP
8. AACVPR
9. Aerobics
10. USOC
11. FIMS

Key Concepts - Review your lecture notes and the textbook. You should be able to answer the following questions:

- ◆ Which professionals will benefit from the study of exercise physiology?

- ◆ How has the general approach to studying the human body changed within the field of exercise physiology over the past 50 years?

- ◆ What is the difference between exercise physiology and kinesiology?

- ◆ What areas does sports medicine encompass?

- ◆ What was the major contribution of each of the following indivduals?

  - ‣ Lavoisier
  - ‣ R. Tait McKenzie
  - ‣ A.V. Hill
  - ‣ D.B. Dill
  - ‣ Arthur Steinhaus
  - ‣ Leonard Larson
  - ‣ Peter Karpovich
  - ‣ Josephine Rathbone
  - ‣ Thomas Cureton
  - ‣ Kenneth Cooper

For each date and name listed, indicate the associated historical event:

1996 -   ACSM & NCPPA (USA) -_____

1996 -   US Surgeon General -   _____

1990s - Applications to health -   _____

1980s - Athletes, rehabilitation -   _____

1970s - Era of rapid expansion -   _____

1968 -   Kenneth Cooper -   _____

1954 -   ACSM (USA) -   _____

1953 -   Kraus & Hirschland -   _____

1940s - WW II -   _____

1930s - A.V. Hill, August Krogh

       & Otto Meyerhof -   _____

1927 - L.J. Henderson

       & D.B. Dill -   _____

1923 - A.V. Hill (England) -   _____

1913 - Benedict & Cathcart -   _____

1894 - Rubner -   _____

1850 - 1890 -Golden era -   _____

1847 - von Helmholtz -   _____

1789 – Lavoisier -   _____

Post Test

Multiple choice

1. The largest, most influencial sports medicine group in the world is
   a. NATA
   b. ACSM
   c. AWHP
   d. AAHPERD

2. The first exercise physiology experiment was conducted by
   a. Dill
   b. Lavoisier
   c. Cooper
   d. Atwater

3. The first studies on anaerobic performance were conducted by
   a. Hill
   b. Cooper
   c. Lavoisier
   d. Atwater

4. Which of the following did not receive a nobel prize for work on muscular studies?
   a. Hill
   b. Meyerhof
   c. Cooper
   d. Krogh

5. A fatigue lab was established in 1927 at which American university?
   a. Princeton
   b. Yale
   c. Rutgers
   d. Harvard

6. The onset of World War I shifted the emphasis of research towards
   a. anaerobic events
   b. fine motor skills
   c. manual dexterity
   d. physical fitness

7. Following World War I the focus of research shifted towards
   a. anaerobic events
   b. rehabilitation
   c. physical fitness
   d. fine motor skills

8. Several professional organizations began publishing _____ which increased their acceptance as academic disciplines.
   a. magazines
   b. newsletters
   c. monographs
   d. journals

9. _____ is often credited with initiating the modern "aerobics craze."
   a. Hill
   b. Cooper
   c. Karpovich
   d. Rathbone

10. The scientific study of human movement is
    a. kinesiology
    b. exercise physiology
    c. sports medicine
    d. biology

Answers - Chapter 1

Pretest

1. B
2. C
3. A
4. D
5. B
6. C
7. A
8. D
9. B

Post Test

1. B
2. B
3. A
4. C
5. D
6. D
7. D
8. D
9. B
10. A

CHAPTER 2
ENERGY SOURCES

Lecture Preparation: Multiple Choice

Instructions: After reading the chapter, read each question and the answer choices. Select the choice which BEST answers the question. Check your answers at the back of this chapter, and review any incorrectly answered questions in your textbook.

Pretest

1. During a track event, a 2-mile run competitor is going to rely primarily on
   a. anaerobic system
   b. aerobic system
   c. ATP-PC system
   d. a blend of anaerobic and aerobic metabolism

2. During resting conditions, about two-thirds of the food fuel is contributed by
   a. protein
   b. carbohydrates
   c. fats
   d. carbohydrates and fats

3. To perform physiological work, humans rely on the transformation of
   a. solar energy to electrical energy
   b. chemical energy to electrical energy
   c. chemical energy to mechanical energy
   d. nuclear energy to solar energy

4. At rest, traces of lactic acid are always present at a constant level, indicative of
   a. LDH converting pyruvate to lactate in anaerobic conditions
   b. LDH converting pyruvate to lactate in aerobic conditions
   c. lack of LDH present at rest and aerobic conditions
   d. decreased efficiency of LDH at rest

5. Which of the following is/are true of ATP?
   I.   it is stored in all muscle cells
   II. it is the immediate source of energy for muscular contraction
   III. ADP can react to form ATP + AMP when catalyzed by the enzyme myokinase
   IV. PC + ADP can form ATP + C when catalyzed by the enzyme creatine kinase
      a. I only
      b. II, III, & IV
      c. I, II, III, & IV
      d. none of the above

6. Low intensities of work which are long in duration will derive ATP from
   a. aerobic glycolysis
   b. Krebs Cycle
   c. the electron transport system
   d. all of the above

7. One of the key regulating enzymes for anaerobic glycolysis is
   a. isocitrate dehydrogenase
   b. phosphorylase
   c. hexokinase
   d. phosphofructokinase

8. Beta oxidation is used in
   a. protein metabolism after the Krebs Cycle
   b. carbohydrate metabolism in preparation for the Krebs Cycle
   c. fat metabolism in preparation for the Krebs Cycle
   d. fat metabolism after the Krebs Cycle

9. Aerobic metabolism occurs
   a. in the cytoplasm
   b. in the mitochondria
   c. both a & b
   d. neither a nor b

10. The end product of the electron transport system is
    a. water & ATP
    b. lactic acid & ATP
    c. water & lactic acid
    d. hydrogen & ATP

11. Before pyruvic acid can enter the Krebs Cycle, it loses CO_2 because it is a
    a. 3-carbon molecule and must be converted to acetyl-CoA which is a 2-carbon molecule
    b. 4-carbon molecule and must be converted to lactic acid which is a 3-carbon molecule
    c. 3-carbon molecule and must be converted to acetyl-CoA which is a 4-carbon molecule
    d. none of the above

12. The electron carriers of ETS contain iron (Fe^{++}) and are referred to as
    a. oxidative enzymes
    b. hemoglobin
    c. cytochomes
    d. mitochondria

13. When one shifts from a steady level of oxygen consumption to a higher one where aerobic metabolism needs to increase to meet the ATP required, this adjustment is referred to as
    a. steady state
    b. oxygen debt
    c. oxygen deficit
    d. none of the above

14. Fatigue during anaerobic glycolysis is likely due to
    I. an increase in lactic acid production beyond removal
    II. inhibition of the rate limiting enzyme
    III. an increase in intracellular pH
    IV. a drop in intracellular pH
        a. I & III only
        b. II & III only
        c. I, II, & IV
        d. I, II, III, & IV

Key Terms - Define the following terms:

1. Energy
2. First Law of Thermodynamics
3. Second Law of Thermodynamics
4. Entropy
5. Redox
6. NAD
7. FAD
8. Posphocreatine
9. Glycolysis
10. Krebs Cycle
11. Electron Transport System
12. VO_2 max
13. Lactate threshold
14. Enzyme
15. Beta oxidation
16. Gluconeogenesis
17. Glycogenesis
18. Endergonic
19. Exergonic
20. Coupled reaction
21. Free energy
22. Respiration
23. Lactate
24. Cytochromes

Key Enzymes - Describe the role of these enzymes by indicating the following:

A. The metabolic pathway it helps control

B. The immediate reaction which it catalyzes

♦ Creatine Kinase

♦ Phosphofructokinase

♦ Lactate Dehydrogenase

♦ Pyruvate Dehydrogenase

♦ Citrate Synthase

♦ Succinate Dehydrogenase

♦ Phosphorylase

♦ Glycogen Synthase

♦ cAMP

Key Concepts - Review your lecture notes and the textbook. You should be able to answer the following questions:

♦ For each energy system, describe where it occurs within the cell.

♦ How do the energy producing capacities for the various systems compare to one another?

♦ What is the difference between pyruvate and lactate?

♦ Why is oxygen required to produce most of our energy?

♦ Why are enzymes critical for energy production?

♦ Describe the various conditions which turn on or turn off glycolysis and gluconeogenesis.

♦ What is meant by hormone amplification?

♦ What is the difference between substrate level and oxidative phosphorylation?

♦ What substances are considered phosphagens?

♦ The energy state of a cell is indicated by levels of which substances?

♦ How are work, power, and energy related?

♦ How can knowledge of the energy systems be used to plan training programs for various sports?

♦ How do males and females compare in regards to energy production and utilization?

Fill in the blank lines to complete the diagram.

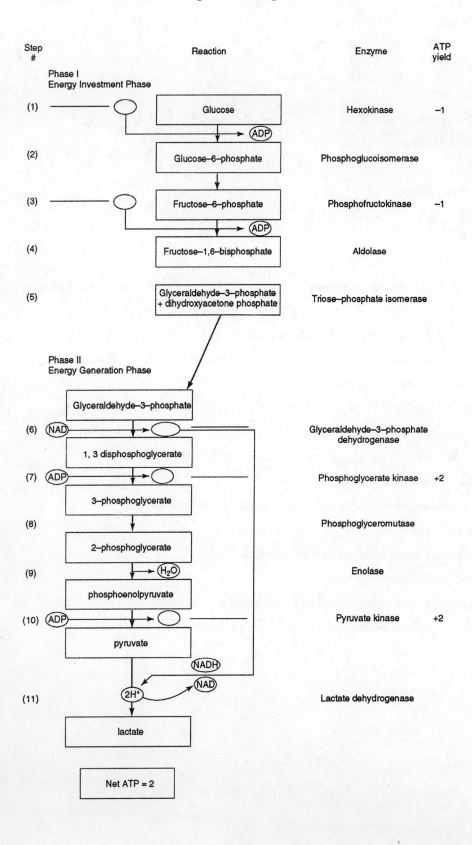

Step #	Reaction	Enzyme	ATP yield

Phase I
Energy Investment Phase

(1) ——— ◯ | Glucose | Hexokinase | −1

→ ADP

(2) | Glucose–6–phosphate | Phosphoglucoisomerase |

(3) ——— ◯ | Fructose–6–phosphate | Phosphofructokinase | −1

→ ADP

(4) | Fructose–1,6–bisphosphate | Aldolase |

(5) | Glyceraldehyde–3–phosphate + dihydroxyacetone phosphate | Triose–phosphate isomerase |

Phase II
Energy Generation Phase

Glyceraldehyde–3–phosphate

(6) NAD ——→ ◯ | 1, 3 disphosphoglycerate | Glyceraldehyde–3–phosphate dehydrogenase |

(7) ADP ——→ ◯ | 3–phosphoglycerate | Phosphoglycerate kinase | +2

(8) | 2–phosphoglycerate | Phosphoglyceromutase |

(9) → H_2O | phosphoenolpyruvate | Enolase |

(10) ADP ——→ ◯ | pyruvate | Pyruvate kinase | +2

NADH
NAD

(11) 2H+ | lactate | Lactate dehydrogenase |

Net ATP = 2

10

Fill in the blank lines to complete the diagram.

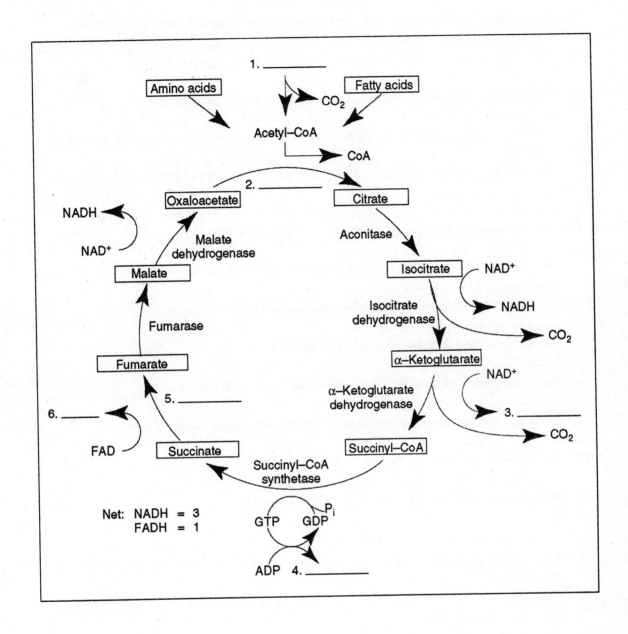

Post Test - Fill in the blank

1. The metabolic process which involves the breakdown of food into water and carbon dioxide.
   _____

2. The amount of heat required to raise one kilogram of water one degree Celsius.
   _____

3. The type of bond which links the final two phosphate groups together within ATP.
   _____

4. The process which partially oxidizes glucose to yield two pyruvate molecules, 2 ATP, and NADH.
   _____

5. The process in which creatine phosphate donates a phosphate to ADP to yield ATP.
   _____

6. The process in which acetyl-CoA molecules combine with oxaloacetate and undergo a series of steps including oxidation and decarboxylation to yield oxaloacetate, NADH, FADH2, ATP, and CO_2 molecules. _____

7. The functional linking of energy released from one reaction to a second energy absorbing reaction.
   _____

8. The final "common pathway" for carbohydrates, fats, and protein oxidation.
   _____

9. The collective name for substances such as PC and ATP.
   _____

10. Protein compounds which accelerate the rate of specific chemical reactions.
    _____

11. Enzymes which commonly regulate phosphorylation or dephosphorylation reactions.
    _____

12. The enzyme which drives the reaction: ADP + ADP -----> ATP + AMP.
    _____

13. The enzyme which drives the reaction: PC + ADP -----> ATP + C.
    _____

14. The storage form of glucose in the human body. _____

15. The names for lactic acid and pyruvic acid after they have dissociated hydrogen ions into their surrounding fluid. _____

16. The enzyme which drives the conversion of pyruvic acid to lactic acid or lactic acid to pyruvic acid.
    _____

17. Two important hydrogen carriers within glycolysis and the Krebs Cycle.
    _____

18. The enzyme which drives the conversion of glycogen to glucose 1-phosphate.
    _____

19. The enzyme which speeds the conversion of glucose to glucose 1-phosphate.
    _____

20. The enzyme considered the "gatekeeper" of glycolysis. It controls the rate of fructose 6-phosphate conversion to fructose 1,6-bisphosphate. _____

21. When a compound accepts a hydrogen and its associated electron.
    _____

22. When a compound donates a hydrogen and its associated electron.

    _____

23. The cellular organelle responsible for the majority of ATP production.

    _____

24. The speed or rate of glycolysis will_____ when there is a high ratio of NADH/NAD+ and FADH$_2$/FAD.

25. The process where long chain fatty acids are broken down into 2 carbon, acetyl groups.

    _____

Multiple Choice - Select the answer which is the best choice.

1.   When a substance loses an electron, it
        a. becomes an acid   b. is reduced
        c. becomes a base   d. is oxidized

2.   NAD and FAD help produce energy by
        a. intercepting hydrogens   b. oxidizing hydrogens
        c. oxidizing carbohydrates   d. reducing carbohydrates

3.   The beginning and ending products of glycolysis may be
        a. glucose-pyruvate   b. glycogen-pyruvate
        c. glucose-lactate   d. a, b, and c

4.   The body stores most of its potential energy as
        a. glucose   b. glycogen
        c. fat   d. protein

5.   Glycolysis takes place
        a. in the mitochondria   b. in the cytosol
        c. in the liver only   d. after beta oxidation

6.   The First law of Thermodynamics explains which of the following?
        a. energy is created by work   b. energy is created in ETS
        c. energy forms are transferred d. ATP is good energy

7.   The Second law of Thermodynamics explains which of the following?
        a. endergonic reactions go naturally   b. an increase in entropy
        c. exergonic RXNs require energy   d. a and b

8.   The energy system(s) with the greatest production capacity
        a. glycolysis   b. Krebs Cycle (alone)
        c. ATP-PC and glycolysis   d. Krebs and ETS

9.   An important enzyme for regulating the rate of glycolysis
        a. phosphofructokinase   b. isocitrate dehydrogenase
        c. succinate dehydrogenase   d. pyruvate dehydrogenase

10.   Fat can be oxidized in the Krebs Cycle following
        a. alpha ketoglutarate   b. anaerobic glycolysis
        c. beta oxidation   d. aerobic glycolysis

11.   Lactate is an end product of
        a. anaerobic glycolysis   b. the Krebs Cycle
        c. the electron transport system d. both a & c

12. Most ATP is actually synthesized during
    a. Krebs Cycle   b. ETS
    c. Glycolysis   d. ATP-PC
13. One mole of glucose is equal to _____ grams
    a. 36   b. 180
    c. 6 x 1023   d. 4
14. The phosphorylation of ADP to yield ATP always involves
    a. an enzyme   b. oxygen
    c. water   d. PC
15. When energy released from one reaction is available to do work it is considered
    a. high energy   b. free energy
    c. kinetic   d. potential
16. The reformation of PC occurs
    a. only during maximal exercise   b. only during low energy states
    c. during recovery from exercise   d. only after creatine supplementation
17. ATP and PC are stored
    a. within the muscle   b. only in the mitochondria
    c. bound to the cell membrane   d. within the cytochromes
18. Beta oxidation occurs
    a. in the mitochondria   b. in the cytosol
    c. only in muscle cells   d. only in the liver
19. The beginning and ending substrates for the Krebs Cycle are
    a. pyruvate-oxaloacetate   b. acetyl-CoA - citrate
    c. pyruvate- citrate   d. oxaloacetate, acetyl-CoA - oxaloacetate
20. The process of beta oxidation produces
    a. one NADH & one FADH2   b. one ATP
    c. an acetyl CoA   d. both a & b
21. Protein contribution to energy production during moderate exercise is estimated to be
    a. 5 - 10%   b. 65 - 70%
    c. 50 - 60%   d. 35 - 50%
22. Proteins enter energy production pathways as
    a. amino acids   b. fatty acids
    c. complex carbohydrates   d. ketones
23. Oxygen is required for _____ to occur
    a. glycolysis   b. ATP-PC
    c. substrate level phosphorylation   d. ETS
24. Short term, very high intensity exercise is predominantly supplied ATP by
    a. Aerobic glycolysis   b. ATP-PC
    c. ETS   d. Krebs Cycle
25. The second messenger, cAMP is responsible for
    a. hormone amplification   b. down regulation
    c. hormone dampening   d. negative feedback

Answers - Chapter 2

Pretest

1. D
2. C
3. C
4. B
5. C
6. D
7. D
8. C
9. B
10. A
11. A
12. C
13. C
14. C

Key Enzymes

Creatine Kinase
a. ATP-PC
b. ADP + CP -->ATP + C

PFK
a. Glycolysis
b. fructose 6P --> fructose 1,6 bisphosphate

LDH
a. Glycolysis
b. pyruvate <---> lactate

PDH
a. Glycolysis to Krebs
b. pyruvate--> acetyl-CoA

Citrate Synthase
a. Krebs Cycle
b. oxaloacetate+ acetyl-CoA --> citrate

SDH
a. Krebs Cycle
b. succinate --> fumarate

Phosphorylase
a. Glycogenolysis
b. Glycogen-->glucose 1P

Glycogen synthase

a. Glycogenesis

b. glucose 1P --> glycogen

cAMP

a. Many RXNs

b. Hormone amplification

Post Test

Fill in the blank

1. oxidation

2. kilocalorie

3. high energy

4. aerobic glycolysis

5. ATP-PC

6. Krebs cycle

7. coupled RXN

8. Krebs Cycle

9. phosphagens

10. enzymes

11. kinases

12. myokinase

13. creatine kinase

14. glycogen

15. lactate, pyruvate

16. LDH

17. NAD & FAD

18. phosphorylase

19. glycogen synthase

20. PFK

21. reduction

22. oxidation

23. mitochondria

24. decrease

25. beta oxidation

Multiple Choice

1. D
2. C
3. D
4. C
5. B
6. C
7. B
8. D
9. A
10. C
11. A
12. B
13. B
14. A
15. B
16. C
17. A
18. A
19. D
20. C
21. A
22. A
23. D
24. B
25. A

CHAPTER 3
RECOVERY FROM EXERCISE

Lecture Preparation: Multiple Choice

Instructions: After reading the chapter, read each question and the answer choices. Select the choice which BEST answers the question. Check your answers at the back of this chapter, and review any incorrectly answered questions in your textbook.

Pretest

1. Following exercise, the length of time in which oxygen consumption remains at a relatively high level depends on

    a. intensity and duration of the bout of exercise

    b. only the duration of the bout of exercise

    c. only the amount of glycogen depleted

    d. only the amount of lactic acid produced

2. The fact that a significant amount of muscle glycogen is resynthesized in 30 minutes to 2 hours following intermittent exercise, and an insignificant amount following continuous exercise is likely due to

    a. more glycogen is depleted during continuous than during intermittent

    b. following intermittent exercise there are a greater amount of glycogen precursors available

    c. the predominant muscle fiber type used in intermittent exercise is faster at glycogen resynthesis

    d. all of the above

3. The fast component of recovery oxygen refers to

    I.   the rapid increase in oxygen consumption in the first 2 to 3 minutes of recovery

    II. the recovery oxygen required solely for the increased temperature effects on metabolism

    III. the recovery concerned with the replenishment of phosphagens (ATP and PC)

    a. I only

    b. II only

    c. III only

    d. I, II, & III

4. The slow component of recovery oxygen refers to

    I.   the gradual decline of oxygen consumption to a resting value

    II. the recovery mainly concerned with the increased temperature effects on metabolism

    III. the recovery concerned with the replenishment of phosphagens (ATP and PC)

    a. I only

    b. I & II only

    c. I & III only

    d. II & III only

5. The duration of rest-recovery needed for the removal of most of the lactic acid from the blood and muscle following exhausting exercise is

    a. approximately 24 to 48 hours   b. approximately 1 hour

    c. approximately 12 to 24 hours   d. less than 3 minutes

6. _____is generally the time needed to replenish ATP and PC phosphagen stores
   a. 2 to 5 minutes of rest-recovery   b. 30 minutes of rest-recovery
   c. 12 hours of rest-recovery   d. 24 hours of rest-recovery

7. The role of the complex protein compound myoglobin is
   a. to serve as a muscular store for oxygen
   b. to serve as a transport of oxygen from the capillaries to the mitochondria
   c. all of the above
   d. none of the above

8. The fastest way in which lactic acid can be removed from the blood and muscles following exhausting exercise is
   a. by stopping the exercise completely and resting
   b. by performing intermittent exercise as a warm down
   c. by performing continuous exercise as a warm down
   d. all of the above are equally effective

9. Myoglobin stores are important during intermittent exercise due to
   a. their size
   b. their rapid restoration with O_2 during recovery
   c. both a & b
   d. their color

10. Which of the following accurately describe possible fates of lactate?
    a. excreted in the urine   b. oxidized to CO_2 and H_2O
    c. converted to glucose   d. all of these answers

Key Terms - Define the following terms:

1. EPOC
2. Recovery oxygen
3. Half reaction time
4. Myoglobin
5. Hemoglobin
6. Q10 effect
7. Gluconeogenesis
8. Lactate
9. Rest-recovery
10. Exercise-recovery

Key Concepts - Review your lecture notes and the textbook. You should be able to answer the following questions:

- Why does oxygen consumption remain elevated above resting levels during recovery from exercise?

- Why are the terms recovery oxygen or EPOC preferable to oxygen debt?

- How does the volume of recovery oxygen change following aerobic exercise training?

- Differentiate between the slow and rapid components of recovery.

- Why is fat replenishment omitted from the list of requirements for recovery oxygen?

- Why is lactate not accurately described as a waste product?

- What are the primary factors determining the length of time required to replenish muscle glycogen stores following exercise?

- Describe the type of food an athlete should consume immediately following exhaustive aerobic exercise, and over the next 24-48 hours.

- What are the roles of myoglobin?

- What occurs during gluconeogenesis?

Post Test

Multiple choice

1. Restoration of muscle phosphagen stores requires
    a. several hours
    b. several days
    c. a few minutes
    d. a high carbohydrate diet

2. The term oxygen debt is currently
    a. being replaced by EPOC
    b. used instead of EPOC
    c. the favored term
    d. both b & c

3. The fast component of recovery includes oxygen fueling the post exercise energy needs of
    a. reducing phosphagens
    b. replacing phosphagens
    c. reducing heart rate
    d. replacing fat deposits

4. The resynthesis of _____ occurs directly as a result of the oxidation of food
    a. PC
    b. fatty acids
    c. muscle glycogen
    d. ATP

5. The replenishment of muscle glycogen does NOT depend upon
    a. type of depletion exercise
    b. amount of carbohydrate in the diet
    c. amount of protein in the diet
    d. availability of glycogen precursors

6. Glycogen resynthesis is most rapid in _____ type of muscle fibers
    a. slow twitch-oxidative
    b. fast twitch-oxidative, glycolytic
    c. fast twitch-glycolytic
    d. there is no difference

7. Lactate is the proper term used to describe the _____ form of Lactic acid
    a. deoxygenated
    b. ionized
    c. reduced
    d. deactivated

8. Lactate concentration immediately following exercise is influenced by
    a. exercise intensity only
    b. exercise duration only
    c. exercise mode only
    d. exercise intensity and duration

9. To optimally remove lactate from working muscles, the average athlete should recover from exercise by
    a. sitting down
    b. performing intermittent exercise
    c. walking slowly
    d. performing moderate exercise

10. The majority of lactate removed from working muscle by the blood is
    a. excreted in the urine
    b. converted to protein
    c. converted to glycogen
    d. oxidized to CO_2 & H_2O

11. The role of myoglobin is to
    a. provide the liver with O_2
    b. facilitate the diffusion of O_2
    c. facilitate the removal of CO_2
    d. store CO_2

12. Plasma FFA levels are _____ immediately following exercise
    a. extremely low
    b. elevated
    c. returned to resting levels
    d. first b, then a

13. Which of the following is NOT a major metabolite for gluconeogenesis?
    a. alanine
    b. tryptophan
    c. pyruvate
    d. lactate

14. The amount of lactate found within the blood at any given time is dependent upon the rate of its
    a. production
    b. excretion
    c. degradation
    d. both a & c
15. During the first 24 hours of recovery from exercise, the carbohydrate source should be
    a. primarily simple sugars
    b. primarily complex carbohydrates
    c. a 50 - 50 combination of a & b
    d. the type of sugar doesn't matter

Answers - Chapter 3

Pretest

1. A
2. D
3. C
4. B
5. B
6. A
7. C
8. C
9. B
10. A, B, C

Post Test

Multiple choice

1. C
2. A
3. B
4. D
5. C
6. C
7. B
8. D
9. D
10. D
11. B
12. B
13. B
14. D
15. D

CHAPTER 4
MEASUREMENT OF ENERGY, WORK, AND POWER

Lecture Preparation: Multiple Choice

Instructions: After reading the chapter, read each question and the answer choices. Select the choice which BEST answers the question. Check your answers at the back of this chapter, and review any incorrectly answered questions in your textbook.

Pretest

1. Measuring O_2 consumption and CO_2 expired, the respiratory exchange ratio (R) represents

    a. VO_2/VCO_2 determined during maximal conditions

    b. VO_2/VCO_2 determined during steady state conditions

    c. VCO_2/VO_2 determined during maximal conditions

    d. VCO_2/VO_2 determined during steady state conditions

2. Energy is described as

    a. the capacity to perform work

    b. force x distance

    c. the ability to perform work in a certain period of time

    d. none of the above

3. Hydrogen reacting with oxygen produces water and 68.4 kcal, and requires 68.4 kcal to break up the water molecule to form hydrogen and water, representing

    a. the principle of the conservation of energy

    b. the application for direct method in the measurement of energy

    c. the first law of thermodynamics

    d. all of the above

4. An exercise "R" of 1.0 would represent

    a. fat oxidation

    b. glucose oxidation

    c. an equal amount of protein, fat and glucose oxidation

    d. low intensity aerobic exercise

5. 1 MET is approximately

    a. the oxygen requirement required to sustain maximal exercise

    b. 3.5 ml × kg-1 × minute-1

    c. both a & b

    d. neither a nor b

6.   Factors that could affect the "R" include
        I.   a person's weight
        II. elevated oxygen consumption during recovery from exercise
        III. a person's intensity level
        IV. the buffering of lactic acid during short-term, exhaustive exercise
            a. I & III only
            b. II & III only
            c. I, II & IV
            d. II, III, & IV

7.   Percent efficiency, physiologically speaking, is measured by
        a. force × distance, divided by time, × 100
        b. kcal of work performed, divided by kcal of energy expended, × 100
        c. kcal of work expended subtracted by the kcal of work performed, × 100
        d. none of the above

8.   Heart rate can be used to estimate oxygen consumption because
        a. there is a linear relationship between oxygen consumption and heart rate response
        b. someone working at a given percentage of maximum heart rate is working at that percentage of VO_2 max
        c. VO_2 max and heart rate max are the exactly the same
        d. all of the above

9.   A person with an exercise "R" of .97
        I.   would have a lower heart rate than if he/she had an "R" of .80
        II. would have a greater rate of lactic acid production than if he/she had an "R" of .80
        III. would have a higher rate of carbohydrate oxidation than if working at a lower heart rate
        IV. would have a higher heart rate than if he/she had an "R" of .80
            a. I only
            b. I, II & III only
            c. II, III & IV only
            d. III, & IV only

10.   Energy expenditure should be expressed relative to body size during
        a. walking
        b. swimming
        c. stationary cycling
        d. both b & c

Key Terms - Define the following terms:

1. Work
2. Power
3. Energy
4. Ergometer
5. Kilocalorie
6. Kilojoule
7. Watt

8. MET

9. Oxygen consumption

10. Respiratory exchange ratio

11. Efficiency

12. Anaerobic power

13. Aerobic power

14. Protocol

Key Concepts - Review your lecture notes and the textbook. You should be able to answer the following questions:

- How are work, power, and energy related?

- How can we directly measure the amount of work an individual performs during exercise?

- How can we indirectly measure the amount of work an individual does during exercise?

- How is the MET used within exercise studies or clinical settings?

- What is the basic mathematical formula for efficiency?

- What does telemetry allow us to do in regards to measuring work?

- What is the difference between anaerobic and aerobic power?

- What is an exercise protocol?

- How can one's respiratory exchange ratio be determined?

- What basic information does the respiratory exchange ratio provide?

Calculating MET Values

Use the following instructions to calculate your 1 MET value. This information can then be used to estimate the number of kcals you utilize each minute, while performing a variety of activities. A sample of these activities may be found on the next page.

1 MET = 3.5 ml oxygen x kg body weight-1 x minute-1

1 Liter of oxygen is roughly equivalent to 5 kcals

Steps:

1. Your current weight in pounds_____
   To get your current weight in kg divide this weight by 2.2
   _____lbs / 2.2 = _____kg

2. To get ml/min multiply 3.5 ml × your weight in kg
   3.5 × _____kg = _____ml × min-1

3. To convert ml × min-1 to L × min-1, divide by 1,000
   _____ml × min-1 / 1,000 = _____L × min-1

4. To get kcals × min-1, multiply L × min-1 by 5
   _____L × min-1 × 5 = _____kcals × min-1

5. Your 1 MET value is equal to the calculated kcals × min-1

6. To determine the number of kcals expended at various MET levels, multiple the number of kcals each minute (as calculated in #4) by the number of METs related to the specific activity.

25

Estimated MET Equivalents for Various Activities

Using your kcal equivalent for 1 MET level of activity as calculated on the previous page, determine the number of kcals you would expend while performing the following activities. To calculate kcals × min-1, multiple your 1 MET kcal equivalent by the MET level in the left hand column.

MET Level		kcals × min-1	Types of activities
0.85 MET	=	_____	Sleeping
1.00 MET	=	_____	Awake, post-absorptive sitting
1.50 METs	=	_____	Standing activities, dressing, showering, light housework
2.00 METs	=	_____	Walking ~1 mph., cycling ~6 mph., Volleyball, sailing, bowling, Heavy housework
3.00 METs	=	_____	Walking ~2.5 mph., tennis doubles, Cycling ~8 mph., Badminton singles ,Ballet, rapid calisthenics
4.00 METs	=	_____	Walking ~4 mph., cycling ~9 mph., Skating, gardening
5.00 METs	=	_____	Walking ~5 mph., cycling ~10 mph. Tennis singles, downhill skiing
6.00 METs	=	_____	Jogging ~5.5 mph., paddle ball, Cycling ~11 mph., Mt. climbing, Ice hockey
7.00 METs	=	_____	Running ~6 mph., racquetball, Cycling ~ 12 mph., handball
8.00 METs	=	_____	Running ~6.5 mph., Cycling ~13 mph.
9.00 METs	=	_____	Running ~7 mph. Cycling ~ 14 mph.
10.0 METs	=	_____	Running ~8 mph.

(These values are estimates. Actual values will vary depending upon efficiency of movement and other conditions such as temperature)

Multiply your calculated kcal values for 1 MET, by each of the listed MET levels to estimate the kcals expended each minute while performing the various activities.

Post Test

Multiple choice

1. The ability to do work
   a. power
   b. force
   c. energy
   d. kilocalorie

2. The formula work / time best describes
   a. power
   b. force
   c. energy
   d. kilocalorie

3. The metabolic equivalent which is estimated at 3.5 ml per kilogram per minute
   a. kilocalorie
   b. MET
   c. kilojoule
   d. calorie

4. The relationship between oxygen consumption and carbon dioxide production reveals
   a. the total amount of work
   b. the net amount of work
   c. type of fuel being oxidized
   d. total power output

5. An indirect method for measuring energy expenditure involves calculating
   a. VO_2 consumption
   b. heat production
   c. efficiency of movement
   d. economy of movement

6. For each liter of oxygen consumed, approximately ____ kcals of energy are available
   a. one
   b. ten
   c. five
   d. these are not related

7. A respiratory exchange ratio of ____ is assumed if it can not be measured
   a. 1.00
   b. 0.83
   c. 0.70
   d. 0.92

8. The benefit of having an "on line" system is
   a. the subject can perform without any equipment
   b. the exercise physiologist can calculate the results while the subject is still exercising
   c. the subject can reach higher performance levels
   d. the exercise physiologist can calibrate their equipment during the exercise trials

9. During steady state exercise the assumption is made that energy is supplied
   a. aerobically
   b. anaerobically
   c. without fat oxidation
   d. without carbohydrate oxidation

10. To calculate the net oxygen cost of an activity one must
    a. subtract resting VO_2 from the total oxygen cost
    b. subtract estimated anaerobic input from the total oxygen cost
    c. subtract resting VO_2 from the steady state value and divide by body weight
    d. subtract the oxygen cost of ventilation from one's resting value

11. Oxygen cost which is expressed for an entire exercise period is a measure of
    a. peak aerobic power
    b. VO_2 max
    c. peak anaerobic power
    d. work

12. The R value can only be determined during
    a. steady state
    b. sleep
    c. intense exercise
    d. the first ten minutes of exercise

13. When fat is oxidized, oxygen is used to combine with
    a. hydrogen, nitrogen, and carbon   b. only hydrogen
    c. both hydrogen and carbon   d. both nitrogen and hydrogen

14. Less energy is available for use when nutrients are oxidized in the body than in a bomb calorimeter due to
    a. water loss   b. nitrogen & sulfur residues are excreted
    c. nitrogen's poor solubility   d. the body doesn't get as hot

15. Measured R values of 1.0 then 0.70 would indicate that ____ & ____ were being oxidized respectively.
    a. protein then fat   b. carbohydrate then fat
    c. protein then carbohydrate   d. fat then carbohydrate

16. With higher intensity activities we would expect to see R values closer to
    a. 0.70   b. 0.83
    c. 0.78   d. 1.00

17. When interpreting R values we must take ____ into consideration
    a. the humidity   b. barometric pressure
    c. wind chill   d. hyperventilation

18. The ratio of work output over work input or energy expenditure × 100 =
    a. respiratory exchange ratio   b. working ratio
    c. economy of movement   d. percent efficiency

19. The velocity achieved for a given rate of oxygen consumed is described as
    a. velocity/O_2 ratio   b. economy of movement
    c. efficiency ratio   d. percent efficiency

20. Which of the following variables is not routinely transmitted via telemetry, during exercise studies?
    a. heart rate   b. body temperature
    c. blood pressure   d. BMI

21. VO2 and heart rate during submaximal exercise are
    a. not related   b. exponentially related
    c. inversely related   d. linearly related

22. At rest, an average individual ventilates about ____ liters of air each minute
    a. 1 - 3   b. 6 - 8
    c. 10 - 12   d. 15 - 20

23. Individual values for oxygen consumption and power output are more useful if expressed
    a. relative to body size or weight   b. relative to their R value
    c. in liters / minute   d. as a percent of expected work output

24. The ability of an individual to produce power in a local muscle site, independent of blood supply
    a. aerobic power   b. peak power
    c. peak work output   d. anaerobic power

25. The measure of one's _____ has both athletic and general public health applications
    a. strength   b. power
    c. cardiorespiratory fitness   d. peak anaerobic power

Answers - Chapter 4

Pretest

1. D
2. A
3. A
4. B
5. B
6. D
7. C
8. A
9. C
10. A

Post Test

Multiple choice

1. C
2. A
3. B
4. C
5. A
6. C
7. B
8. B
9. A
10. A
11. D
12. A
13. B
14. B
15. B
16. D
17. D
18. D
19. B
20. D
21. D
22. B
23. A
24. D
25. C

CHAPTER 5
NERVOUS CONTROL OF MUSCULAR MOVEMENT

Lecture Preparation: Multiple Choice

Instructions: After reading the chapter, read each question and the answer choices. Select the choice which BEST answers the question. Check your answers at the back of this chapter, and review any incorrectly answered questions in your textbook.

Pretest

1. The central nervous system consists of
    a. the brain   b. the spinal cord
    c. the extremities   d. both a & b

2. The learning of a motor skill takes place in the
    a. efferent neurons   b. hypothalamus.
    c. cerebral cortex and cerebellum   d. the proprioceptors

3. The basic functional unit of a nerve is the neuron, which consists of
    a. a cell body, dendrites and axon
    b. a proprioceptor and a cell body
    c. an efferent dendrite, a cell body, and an afferent dendrite
    d. none of the above

4. A neurotransmitter that could elicit a excitatory post synaptic potential (EPSP) at the neuromuscular junction is
    a. gamma-aminobutyric acid (GABA)
    b. glycine
    c. ATP
    d. acetylcholine (ACh)

5. A neurotransmitter that commonly elicits an inhibitory post synaptic potential (IPSP) in the brain is
    a. norepinephrine
    b. gamma-aminobutyic acid (GABA)
    c. serotonin
    d. dopamine

6. Excitatory neurotransmitters increase a cell membrane's permeability to _____, and if the influx is great enough it may lead to _____ of the cell.
    a. potassium (K+)/depolarization
    b. sodium (Na+)/depolarization
    c. potassium (K+)/ hyperpolarization
    d. sodium (Na+)/ hyperpolarization

7. Inhibitory neurotransmitters increase a cell membranes permeability to _____, and leads to
_____.
   a. potassium (K+) and chloride (Cl-)/depolarization
   b. sodium (Na+)/depolarization
   c. potassium (K+) and chloride (Cl-)/ hyperpolarization
   d. sodium (Na+)/hyperpolarization

8. The sequence of the reflex arc consists of
   a. afferent nerve to the spinal cord, efferent nerve to the motor response
   b. afferent nerve to the spinal cord, sensory nerve to the motor response
   c. efferent nerve to the spinal cord, afferent nerve to the motor response
   d. none of the above

9. The group of various muscle sense organs that transmit information about limb position to the central nervous system are the
   a. alpha motor nerves
   b. intrafusal fibers
   c. proprioceptors
   d. annulospiral nerves

10. The most abundant type of proprioceptor which are often referred to as stretch receptors are
   a. golgi tendon organs
   b. muscle spindles
   c. pacinian corpuscles
   d. bulbs of Krause

Key Terms - Define the following terms:

1. Axon
2. Dendrite
3. Cell body
4. Myelin
5. Synapse
6. Action potential
7. Neurotransmitter
8. Norepinephrine
9. Acetylcholine
10. Gamma-amino butyric acid (GABA)
11. Spatial summation
12. Temporal summation
13. Proprioceptors
14. Muscle spindles
15. Golgi tendon organs
16. Alpha-gamma coactivation
17. Reciprocal inhibition

Key Concepts - Review your lecture notes and the textbook. You should be able to answer the following questions:

- ♦ What are the major components of the central nervous system?
- ♦ What role does the central nervous system play in initiating and controlling movement?
- ♦ What are the divisions of the autonomic nervous system?
- ♦ How is an action potential initiated?
- ♦ How are action potentials relayed from one nerve to another?
- ♦ What role do proprioceptors play in controlling movement patterns?
- ♦ What is a reflex arc?
- ♦ How does excitation or inhibition occur at a synapse?
- ♦ Describe the manner in which a voluntary motor skill is performed.
- ♦ What is the role of the cerebellum in controlling movement patterns?
- ♦ What is a motor engram?

Label the following diagram using the words provided in the word bank:

Word Bank

Axon	Dendrite	Cell body	Myelin	Synaptic vesicle
Nucleus	Nucleolus	Nissel bodies	Axon hillock	Presynaptic membrane
Endfoot	Synaptic cleft	Acetylcholine	Receptor	Postsynaptic membrane

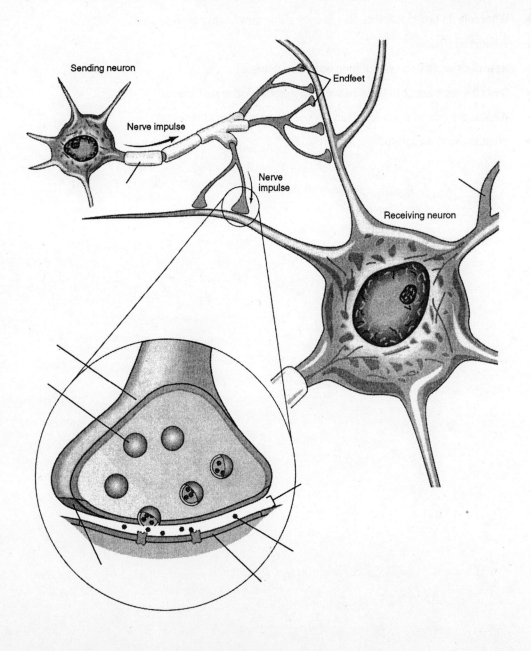

Post Test

Multiple choice

1. The central nervous system is composed of the
   - a. cerebellum & cerebral cortex
   - b. brain & spinal cord
   - c. thalamus & hypothalamus
   - d. pons & medulla

2. The branch of the autonomic nervous system associated with increasing the metabolic activity of most body systems
   - a. parasympathetic
   - b. sensory
   - c. motor
   - d. sympathetic

3. The portion of a nerve which carries a stimuli towards the cell body
   - a. soma
   - b. myelin sheath
   - c. axon
   - d. dendrite

4. The portion of a nerve which carries an action potential away from the cell body
   - a. soma
   - b. dendrite
   - c. axon
   - d. myelin sheath

5. The speed of the action potential will increase with the presence of
   - a. GABA
   - b. myelin
   - c. glycine
   - d. serine

6. One motor nerve and all of the muscle fibers it innervates is called a
   - a. nerve-fiber unit
   - b. fiber-nerve unit
   - c. functional unit
   - d. motor unit

7. The difference in electrical charge between the inside and outside of a cell establishes the
   - a. osmotic flow
   - b. resting membrane potential
   - c. counter current
   - d. post synaptic flow pattern

8. The neurotransmitter released from vesicles of motor nerves is
   - a. GABA
   - b. glycine
   - c. epinephrine
   - d. acetylcholine

9. A neurotransmitter may be considered excitatory if it increases the membrane's permeability to
   - a. sodium
   - b. calcium
   - c. chloride
   - d. potassium

10. A neurotransmitter is considered inhibitory if it increases a cell membrane's permeability to
    - a. sodium
    - b. potassium
    - c. calcium
    - d. magnesium

11. The additive effect of a various stimuli received within a short time at a synapse is called
    - a. stimuli summation
    - b. spatial summation
    - c. temporal summation
    - d. ionic summation

12. Sensory organs which increase one's kinesthesis are called
    - a. sensory bulbs
    - b. perceptors
    - c. sensory vesicles
    - d. proprioceptors

13. Information regarding the amount of stretch or tension placed on a muscle fiber is sent to the CNS via
    - a. pacinian corpuscles
    - b. muscle spindles
    - c. ruffini endings
    - d. gamma units

14. Large motor nerves which innervate skeletal muscle fibers are classified as _____ fibers.
    a. gamma   b. beta
    c. alpha   d. delta

15. The muscle spindles can activate themselves via the
    a. alpha motor system   b. beta loop
    c. delta motor system   d. gamma loop

16. Resting muscle has a small amount of resistance to stretch. This is referred to as muscle
    a. tone   b. excitability
    c. resistance   d. reflex resistance

17. Activation of Golgi tendon organs results in a _____ within the muscle.
    a. strong reflexive contraction b. weak reflexive contraction
    c. jerky contraction   d. relaxation

18. Which of the following is not a joint receptor
    a. GTO   b. pacinian corpuscle
    c. ruffini end organ   d. bulbs of Krause

19. The following centers are responsible for learning new motor skills
    a. pons & medulla   b. thalamus & hypothalamus
    c. hippocampus & thalamus   d. cerebral cortex & cerebellum

20. Pyramidal cell firing in the brain encodes two aspects of movement
    a. force & direction   b. speed & accuracy
    c. accuracy & direction   d. precision & speed

21. An area of the brain considered the "sports skill area" is composed of the____ & ____ areas.
    a. premotor, postmotor   b. premotor, supplemental motor
    c. supplemental motor, postmotor d. postmotor, presupplemental

22. The is responsible for coordinating movement patterns in large groups of muscles.
    a. cerebral cortex   b. hypothalamus
    c. thalamus   d. cerebellum

23. The cerebellum initiates a "correcting" effect known as
    a. dampening   b. adjusting
    c. neocortical override   d. cerebellum reflex

24. Memorized motor patterns are also called
    a. motorgrams   b. motor memorygrams
    c. motor engrams   d. motor memories

25. Henry's memory drum demonstrates that motor ability is
    a. general   b. task specific
    c. inherited   d. transferable

Answers - Chapter 5

Pretest

1. D
2. C
3. A
4. D

36

5. B
6. B
7. C
8. A
9. C
10. B

Post Test

Multiple choice

1. B
2. D
3. D
4. C
5. B
6. D
7. B
8. D
9. A
10. B
11. C
12. D
13. B
14. C
15. D
16. A
17. D
18. A
19. D
20. A
21. B
22. D
23. A
24. C
25. B

CHAPTER 6
SKELETAL MUSCLE: STRUCTURE AND FUNCTION

Lecture Preparation: Multiple Choice

Instructions: After reading the chapter, read each question and the answer choices. Select the choice which BEST answers the question. Check your answers at the back of this chapter, and review any incorrectly answered questions in your textbook.

1. A high muscle fiber:nerve ratio (F:N ratio) is associated with
    I.   very precise movements
    II. gross movements with high force
    III. low force movements
    IV. precise movements with high force
        a. I only
        b. II only
        c. I & III only
        d. IV only

2. The sarcoplasmic reticulum plays a large role in regulating
    a. nuclei, myofibril and mitochondria
    b. glycogen, PC, and ATP
    c. calcium
    d. all of the above

3. Some researchers believe that fatigue can be caused at the neuromuscular junction due to
    a. decreased release of acetylcholine from a nerve ending, usually involving Type I fibers
    b. decreased action potentials in the sarcolemma of the Type I fibers
    c. decreased release of acetylcholine from a nerve ending, usually involving Type II fibers
    d. none of the above

4. The all-or-none law refers to the fact that
    a. a maximal stimulus contracts all the fibers and a minimal stimulus contracts just one fiber
    b. a stimulus sufficient to contract one fiber, will contract all the fibers of a motor unit
    c. all fibers of a motor unit will contract or none will contract
    d. both b & c

5. Type I fibers are
    a. always recruited regardless of exercise intensity
    b. recruited once fatigue sets in
    c. are slow and are recruited last
    d. both b & c

6. A positive training adaptation in relation to muscle fibers is
    a. possible improved oxidative capacity in all fibers and glycolytic capacity of Type II fibers
    b. possible increased number of Type II fibers
    c. possible increased Type IIc fibers
    d. all of the above

7. Muscles are attached to bone by
   a. ligaments
   b. sarcolemmas
   c. tendons
   d. a direct attachment between muscle fiber and bone
8. With increasing velocities of movement the peak force generated by a muscle
   a. increases
   b. decreases
   c. remains the same
   d. there is no set pattern
9. An isometric or static contraction, provides tension by
   a. visible muscle shortening
   b. ATP cross-bridges being recycled while the actins remain in a relative position
   c. visible muscle lengthening
   d. none of the above
10. Muscle strength gradations are made possible by
    a. varying the frequency of contraction of individual motor units
    b. varying the number of motor units contracting at any given time
    c. by multiple motor unit summation and wave summation
    d. all of the above
11. Type II fibers are very important in
    I.   walking
    II. a javelin throw
    III. a marathon run
    IV. the forty-yard dash
        a. II only
        b. II & IV only
        c. I & III only
        d. II, III & IV
12. Type I fibers are very important in
    I.   walking
    II. a javelin throw
    III. a marathon run
    IV. the forty-yard dash
        a. II only   b. II & III only
        c. I & III only   d. II, III & IV only
13. With a high Type II fiber distribution in the muscle
    a. the peak power is increased and the peak force is decreased
    b. the peak power is increased and the peak force is increased
    c. the peak power is decreased and the peak force is increased
    d. the peak power is decreased and the peak force is decreased

Key Terms - Define the following terms:

1. Myofibril

2. Myofilament

3. Sarcomere

4. Sarcoplasmic reticulum

5. Sliding filament theory

6. Motor unit

7. Henneman's size principle

8. All-or-none law

9. Multiple motor unit summation

10. Wave summation

11. Isoform

12. Hypertrophy

13. Hyperplasia

14. Motor endplate

Key Concepts - Review your lecture notes and the textbook. You should be able to answer the following questions:

- What role does the sarcoplasmic reticulum play in generating a muscle contraction?

- How are muscles attached to bones?

- What is the difference in the number of capillaries surrounding each muscle fiber when comparing a trained versus an untrained individual?

- Describe the role of calcium in generating a muscle contraction.

- Why is ATP required for muscular contraction?

- Describe a motor unit and explain how the all-or-none law applies to these units.

- How is the strength of a muscular contraction graded?

- Describe the functional differences between Type I and Type II muscle fibers.

- What is meant by the size principle?

- What does muscle plasticity refer to?

- Describe the differences between males and females in reference to muscle fiber composition, size, and strength.

- Differentiate between muscle hypertrophy and hyperplasia.

- Explain what occurs during muscular fatigue.

Label the following structures using the words provided in the word bank:

Word Bank

Epimysium	Perimysium	Endomysium	Sarcolemma
Myofibrils	Tendon	Fasciculus	Capillaries
Sarcomere	Neuromuscular junction	Sarcoplasmic reticulum	Nerve fiber

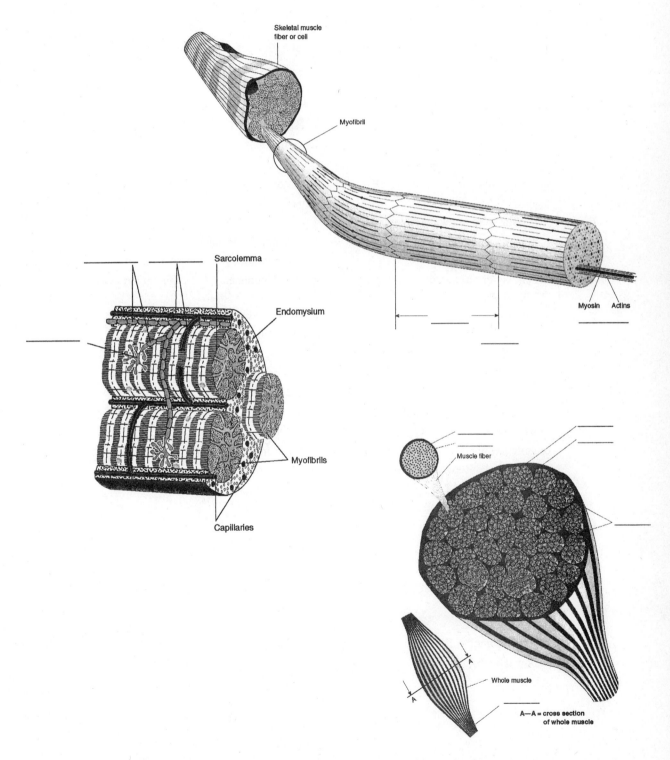

Skeletal muscle fiber or cell

Myofibril

Myosin   Actins

Sarcolemma

Endomysium

Myofibrils

Capillaries

Muscle fiber

Whole muscle

A—A = cross section of whole muscle

Post Test

Multiple Choice

1. The connective tissue surrounding an individual muscle fiber

   a. epimysium   b. perimysium

   c. sarcoplasmic reticulum   d. endomysium

2. The connective tissue which binds several fibers together, forming a fasciculi

   a. epimysium   b. perimysium

   c. sarcoplasmic reticulum   d. endomysium

3. Muscle plasticity refers to the ability of muscle to

   a. contract   b. adaptively change

   c. stretch   d. respond

4. The muscle cell membrane

   a. sarcolemma   b. sarcomere

   c. endomysium   d. perimysium

5. The outermost covering of a bone

   a. perimysium   b. sarcolemma

   c. sarcomere   d. periosteum

6. The point of termination of a motor nerve

   a. ATPase junction   b. neuromuscular junction

   c. sensory endplate   d. motor terminus

7. When two different molecules have the same atomic components, but different structural arrangements

   a. isoforms   b. isostructures

   c. myomere   d. myofibrils

8. The contractile proteins, actin and myosin, may also be called

   a. myofilaments   b. myomeres

   c. myoglobins   d. muscle fibers

9. The functional unit of a skeletal muscle

   a. sarcolemma   b. sarcomere

   c. sarcoplasmic reticulum   d. motor unit

10. The network of tubules and vesicles surrounding the myofibril

    a. sarcomere   b. sarcoplasm

    c. sarcoplasmic reticulum   d. sarcolemma

11. A long thin protein which lies along the surface of the actin strand

    a. myosin   b. troponin

    c. tropo-actin   d. tropomyosin

12. The protein which changes its conformation when calcium binds to it

    a. myosin   b. troponin

    c. tropo-actin   d. tropomyosin

13. An "uncharged" ATP cross-bridge complex is characteristic of _____ muscle.

    a. slow twitch   b. resting

    c. fast twitch   d. active

14. The enzyme, _____ hydrolyzes ATP into ADP and _____
   a. actin ATPase, ADP
   b. myosin ATPase, P_i
   c. actin ATPase, P_i
   d. myosin ATPase, ADP

15. The contractile protein which contains the cross-bridge sites
   a. myosin
   b. troponin
   c. tropo-actin
   d. tropomyosin

16. The type of muscular contraction usually associated with "negative" work
   a. eccentric
   b. isometric
   c. concentric
   d. isokinetic

17. Varying the number of motor units contracting at any one time is referred to as _____ summation.
   a. wave
   b. temporal
   c. multiple motor unit
   d. spatial

18. The variation in proportions of different fiber types in humans is best described as
   a. a very small variation
   b. a great variation
   c. no variation
   d. research hasn't revealed this yet

19. The increase in muscle size due to an increased number of fibers
   a. hyperplasia
   b. hyperplasticity
   c. hypertrophy
   d. atrophy

20. An increase in the size of muscle fibers
   a. hyperplasia
   b. hyperplasticity
   c. hypertrophy
   d. atrophy

21. Sprinters usually have a higher proportion of Type _____ muscle fibers than endurance athletes
   a. I
   b. IIA
   c. IIB
   d. both b & c

22. Which of the following have been identified as potential sites involved in muscular fatigue?
   a. neuromuscular junction
   b. central nervous system
   c. motor nerve
   d. contractile mechanism

23. Lactic acid may contribute to fatigue by inhibiting
   a. PFK
   b. Ca++ -troponin interactions
   c. ATPase
   d. both a & b

24. Motor nerves originate in the
   a. muscles
   b. proprioceptor
   c. spinal area
   d. motor complexes

25. The preferential recruitment of muscle fibers occurs according to the _____ principle.
   a. summation
   b. size
   c. all-or-none
   d. recruitment

For each characteristic listed, indicate whether it is higher in Type I or Type II fibers.

1. Glycogen stores
2. Triglyceride stores
3. PC stores
4. Myoglobin content
5. Oxidative enzymes
6. Capillary density
7. Physical size or diameter

8. Myosin ATPase activity
9. Glycolytic enzyme activity
10. Fatigue resistance
11. Motoneuron size
12. Force production
13. Elasticity
14. Motoneuron recruitment threshold

Section II - Multiple Choice

1. The physiological principle in which strength and endurance are developed is called
   a. specificity of training
   b. training mode
   c. overload
   d. intensity

2. When a muscle shortens while lifting a constant load, the tension developed depends on
   a. the speed of the shortening
   b. the angle of pull
   c. the length of the muscle
   d. all of the above

3. The law of specificity is applied to improve the strength or endurance of a certain skill if
   I. the program includes exercises for the muscle groups the skill involves
   II. the program includes sufficient cross training for recovery
   III. the program includes exercises that simulate the motor patterns the skill involves
   IV. the program is performed with a specific frequency
      a. I & III only
      b. I & IV only
      c. I , III, & IV only
      d. I, II, III, & IV

4. Flexibility is
   a. related to health
   b. possibly related to athletic performance
   c. the range of motion in a joint
   d. all of the above

5. At 60% of its resting length, the tension a muscle develops is near zero because
   a. the actin filaments are pulled completely out of the range of the cross-bridges
   b. there is a overlap of actin filaments so that the filament from one side interferes with the coupling potential of the other side
   c. the angle of pull is such that optimum tension is reduced
   d. all of the above

6. The training principle which pertains to providing adequate time to rest
   a. recovery
   b. reversibility
   c. progression
   d. overload

7. Isotonic contractions using constant loads are at a disadvantage because
   a. the heaviest weight that can be lifted is that which can be lifted at the weakest angle of pull
   b. at certain joint angles the muscle will not be exerting tension near its maximal force
   c. maximum tension can not be distributed completely through the range of motion
   d. all of the above

8. Hypertrophy of muscle fibers can be attributed to
   I. increased number and size of myofibrils per muscle fiber
   II. increased capillary density per muscle fiber
   III. increased total amount of contractile protein, particularly the myosin filament
   IV. increased amount and strength of connective tissues
      a. I only
      b. I & III only
      c. I, II & III only
      d. I, II, III & IV

9. When tension is developed without a change in external length of the muscle
   a. an isokinetic contraction is being performed
   b. an isometric contraction is being performed
   c. a concentric contraction is being performed
   d. an eccentric contraction is being performed

10. Skeletal muscle changes that have been proven to occur in response to resistance training programs are
   a. interconversion of fast-twitch and slow-twitch fibers and decrease in Type II:Type I fiber area
   b. increases in concentrations of creatine, PC, ATP and glycogen within the muscle
   c. an increase in mitochondria density and ATP turnover enzyme activities (e.g. myokinase)
   d. all of the above

11. The following is true concerning delayed onset muscular soreness
   I. it is pain that develops 24 to 48 hours following a bout of exercise
   II. it is most pronounced following eccentric muscular contractions
   III. it is most likely due to damaged connective tissues
   IV. stretching, proper progression and vitamin C intake, have all been suggested to possibly reduce the likelihood and/or severity of muscular soreness
      a. I & III only
      b. II and III only
      c. I, II & III only
      d. I, II, III & IV

12. The Valsalva maneuver is
   a. attempted expiration against a closed glottis (opening between the vocal cords)
   b. dangerous, as it causes a rise in intrathoracic pressures resulting in a rise in blood pressure
   c. common with isometric contractions
   d. all of the above

13. The resistance training proven to be most effective in comparative studies for improving strength and muscular endurance is

   a. isokinetic programs

   b. isometric programs

   c. isotonic programs

   d. eccentric programs

14. A plyometric exercise consists of

   a. an isotonic contraction followed by a post stretch

   b. a prestretch followed by an immediate eccentric contraction

   c. a prestretch followed by an immediate concentric contraction

   d. none of the above

15. The potential benefit(s) of a plyometric program is/are

   a. the utilization of the stored elastic energy in a muscle-tendon unit by stimulating muscle spindles

   b. enhanced recruitment of facilitated motor neurons and their associated motor units

   c. improved explosive muscular power

   d. all of the above

16. Proprioceptive neuromuscular facilitation (PNF) is

   a. an effective form of plyometric training

   b. an effective flexibility exercise consisting of an isometric contraction in a final stretch position, followed by relaxation and then repeated

   c. the preferred flexibility exercise to reduce risk of injury

   d. both b & c

Answers - Chapter 6

Pretest

1. B
2. C
3. C
4. D
5. A
6. A
7. C
8. B
9. B
10. D
11. B
12. C
13. B

Post Test

1. D
2. B
3. B
4. A
5. D
6. B
7. A
8. A
9. B
10. C
11. D
12. B
13. B
14. B
15. A
16. A
17. C
18. B
19. A
20. C
21. D
22. A, B, C, D
23. D
24. C
25. B

Fiber Characteristics

1. II
2. I
3. II
4. I
5. I
6. I
7. II
8. II

9. II

10. I

11. II

12. II

13. II

14. II

Section II

Multiple Choice

1. C

2. D

3. A

4. D

5. B

6. A

7. D

8. B

9. B

10. B

11. D

12. D

13. D

14. C

15. D

16. D

CHAPTER 7
PULMONARY VENTILATION AND MECHANICS

Lecture Preparation: Multiple Choice

Instructions: After reading the chapter, read each question and the answer choices. Select the choice which BEST answers the question. Check your answers at the back of this chapter, and review any incorrectly answered questions in your textbook.

1. The tissue surrounding the lungs which serves to protect & lubricate
    a. pleura   b. alveoli
    c. bronchi   d. trachea

2. The categories used to describe various combinations of lung volumes
    a. physiological spaces   b. anatomical spaces
    c. capacities   d. non overlapping volumes

3. The point at which lactate production becomes greater than its removal or clearance
    a. anaerobic threshold   b. steady state threshold
    c. aerobic threshold   d. lactate threshold

4. The total volume of air which a fully inflated lung can hold
    a. residual volume   b. total lung capacity
    c. vital capacity   d. inspiratory reserve volume

5. An instrument used to measure various lung volumes
    a. FEV meter   b. spirometer
    c. spirograph   d. FVC meter

6. Pleura serves to
    a. protect & lubricate   b. increase surface thickness
    c. fight bacteria   d. increase diffusion capacity

7. Smoking cigarettes will _____ the oxygen cost of ventilation
    a. decrease   b. increase
    c. not alter   d. eliminate

8. The technical term for labored breathing
    a. apnea   b. hypoxia
    c. dyspnea   d. sarcopenia

9. The volume of air moved in or out per breath
    a. minute ventilation   b. inspiratory reserve volume
    c. expiratory reserve volume   d. tidal volume

10. The volume of air remaining in the lungs following a maximal exhalation
    a. residual volume   b. inspiratory reserve volume
    c. expiratory reserve volume   d. tidal volume

Key Terms - Define the following terms:

1. Pleura
2. Tidal volume
3. Vital Capacity
4. Minute ventilation
5. Lactate threshold
6. Alveolar ventilation
7. Dyspnea
8. Hyperventilation
9. Spirometer
10. Lung volume
11. Lung capacity

Key Concepts - Review your lecture notes and the textbook. You should be able to answer the following questions:

♦ How does the body maintain a blood pH close to 7.4?

♦ What function do the visceral and parietal pleura perform?

♦ What is meant by getting a second wind?

♦ Explain the mechanism involved in a stitch in the side.

♦ What prevents the lungs from collapsing under normal conditions?

♦ How do lung volumes and capacities compare to one another?

♦ What factors influence the ventilatory rate?

♦ How and why does ventilation change during exercise and recovery?

♦ What factors might influence the rate of lactate production and clearance?

♦ What influence does cigarette smoking have on the oxygen cost of ventilation?

Label the following structures using the words provided in the word bank:

Word Bank

Terminal bronchiole   Larynx   Trachea   Primary bronchus

Alveolar sac   Alveoli   Pharynx   Secondary bronchus

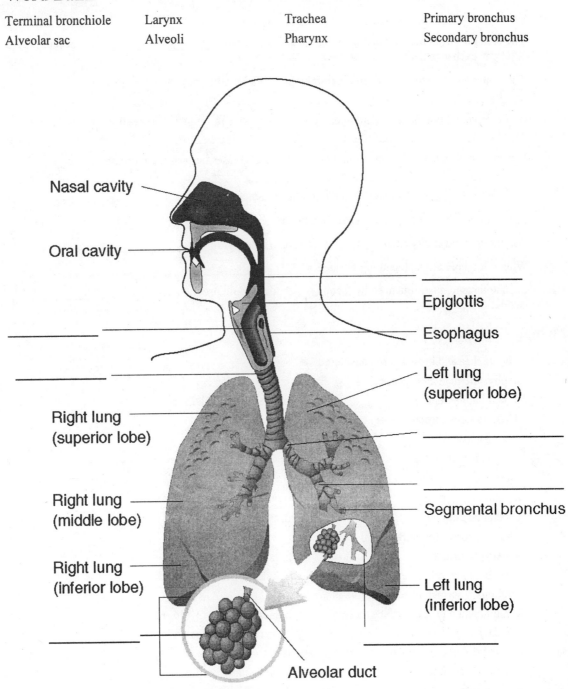

Nasal cavity

Oral cavity

Epiglottis

Esophagus

Left lung
(superior lobe)

Right lung
(superior lobe)

Right lung
(middle lobe)

Segmental bronchus

Right lung
(inferior lobe)

Left lung
(inferior lobe)

Alveolar duct

Post Test

Fill in the blank

1. Expiration is _____ at rest.

2. The area known as the conducting system is also known as _____ because there is no gas exchange here.

3. The volume of air which you can maximally inspire after a normal inhalation is called _____ .

4. Alveolar ventilation is dependent upon ventilatory depth and frequency as well as_____.

5. During exercise, the point where minute ventilation increases beyond the increase in energy demand_____.

6. What are the primary muscles involved in inhalation?_____.

7. Lung volumes are measured with a device known as a _____.

8. The intrapleural cavity enables the lungs to inflate by providing a _____ pressure area.

9. When blood pH drops, breathing frequency _____.

10. Lactate threshold is influenced by factors which affect both production & _____of lactate.

Multiple Choice

1. The trachea and bronchi are considered
   a. physiological dead space
   b. propagation zone
   c. ventilatory zone
   d. anatomical dead space

2. Tidal volume x frequency =
   a. vital capacity
   b. minute ventilation
   c. minute respiration
   d. O_2 cost of ventilation

3. The volume of air which may be expired after a maximal inhalation
   a. total lung capacity
   b. vital capacity
   c. residual volume
   d. tidal volume

4. The function of the intrapleural cavity is to
   a. help O_2 diffuse in
   b. help CO_2 diffuse out
   c. create a low pressure area
   d. balance N_2

5. Pulmonary surfactant serves a role in
   a. maintaining proper surface tension
   b. increasing a-vO_2 difference
   c. decreasing PCO_2
   d. increasing perfusion

6. Inequalities in the ventilation perfusion ratio lead to
   a. wasted ventilation
   b. inadequate perfusion
   c. inadequate ventilation
   d. poor circulation

7. The volume of air in the lungs after a maximal exhalation
   a. residual capacity
   b. residual function
   c. functional residual capacity
   d. residual volume

8. A substance which may accept a H^+
   a. base
   b. acid
   c. free radical
   d. oxidizing agent

9. A substance which can donate a H^+
   a. acid
   b. base
   c. free radical
   d. oxidizing agent

10. Tidal volume x frequency =
    a. vital capacity
    b. minute ventilation
    c. minute respiration
    d. O_2 cost of ventilation

11. The volume of air in the lungs after a maximal inhalation
    a. total lung capacity
    b. vital capacity
    c. residual volume
    d. tidal volume

12. Hyperventilation serves to
    a. maintain proper surface tension
    b. increase a-VO_2 difference
    c. decrease PCO_2
    d. increase perfusion

13. Inequalities in the ventilation perfusion ratio may be caused by
    a. high CO_2 levels
    b. inadequate perfusion
    c. inadequate ventilation
    d. either b or c

14. The volume of air one may expire after a normal exhalation
    a. residual capacity
    b. expiratory reserve volume
    c. functional residual capacity
    d. residual volume

15. The volume of air maximally inspired after a normal inhalation
    a. inspiratory reserve volume
    b. inspiratory capacity
    c. inspiratory volume
    d. vital capacity

16. Lung volumes are
    a. overlapping
    b. non-overlapping
    c. all the same
    d. the cause of V/Q inequalities

17. The mechanism involved in a stitch in the side
    a. ischemia in the diaphragm
    b. increased PO_2
    c. increased PCO_2
    d. intercostal separation

18. Central chemoreceptors responsible for ventilatory drive respond directly to levels of _____
    a. PCO
    b. H^+
    c. 2,3 DPG
    d. bicarbonate

19. The ventilatory response to exercise _____ as a result of training
    a. increases
    b. decreases
    c. stays the same
    d. disappears

20. One indirect method of determining lactate threshold
    a. point of ischemia in the diaphragm
    b. V-slope
    c. CO_2 rebreathing method
    d. point of intercostal separation

21. The respiratory system aids in acid-base balance by altering
    a. rate of ventilation
    b. depth of ventilation
    c. CO_2 levels
    d. all of these answers

22. The alkali reserve refers to the amount of _____ available for buffering
   a. CO
   b. CO_2
   c. pH
   d. HCO_3-
23. The oxygen cost of ventilation is increased by
   a. cigarette smoking
   b. sleeping
   c. increased perfusion
   d. increased capillary density
24. Voluntary hyperventilation produces the following physiological effect
   a. increase oxygen consumption
   b. increase PO_2
   c. decrease anaerobic glycolysis
   d. none of these answers
25. Hypocapnia refers to low
   a. oxygen levels
   b. bicarbonate
   c. blood sugar
   d. CO_2 levels

Answers - Chapter 7

Pretest

1. A
2. C
3. D
4. B
5. B
6. A
7. B
8. C
9. D
10. A

Post Test

Fill in the blank

1. passive
2. anatomical dead space
3. inspiratory reserve volume
4. anatomical dead space
5. hyperventilation
6. diaphragm, external intercostals
7. spirometer
8. low
9. increases
10. clearance

Multiple Choice

1. D
2. B
3. B
4. C
5. A
6. A
7. D
8. A
9. A
10. B
11. A
12. C
13. D
14. B
15. A
16. B
17. A
18. B
19. B
20. B
21. D
22. D
23. A
24. D
25. D

CHAPTER 8
GAS EXCHANGE AND TRANSPORT

Lecture Preparation: Multiple Choice

Instructions: After reading the chapter, read each question and the answer choices. Select the choice which BEST answers the question. Check your answers at the back of this chapter, and review any incorrectly answered questions in your textbook.

1. In the pulmonary capillaries, the PCO_2 decreases and the PO_2 increases due to
    I.   the partial pressure differences between the alveoli and pulmonary capillaries
    II. diffusion of gasses at the alveolar-capillary membrane takes about half the time the blood remains in the pulmonary capillaries
    III. diffusion of gasses at the alveolar-capillary membrane takes about the same time the blood remains in the pulmonary capillaries during intense exercise
    IV. the pressure gradient for PO_2 at the alveolar-capillary membrane is approximately 60 mm Hg and 6 mm Hg for PCO_2, facilitating an increased arterial PO_2 and decreased PCO_2
        a. I only
        b. II & III only
        c. I & IV only
        d. I, II, III & IV

2. Oxygen is transported in the blood in
    a. the hemoglobin (Hgb) molecule to form oxyhemoglobin ($HgbO_2$)
    b. the plasma
    c. both a & b
    d. none of the above

3. In reference to the Oxyhemoglobin Dissociation Curve, a shift to the right indicates
    I.   a possible increase in 2,3 DPG concentration, body temperature, and/or CO_2
    II. a possible decrease in blood pH
    III. a stronger affinity of oxygen to the hemoglobin molecule
    IV. a weaker affinity of oxygen to the hemoglobin molecule
        a. I & III only
        b. I & IV only
        c. I, II & III
        d. I, II & IV

4. The main contributing factor leading to the thirteen fold increase in VO_2 from rest to heavy exercise is
    a. the local adaptations leading to a decreased a-vO_2 difference
    b. an increased blood flow
    c. both a & b are equally important
    d. neither a or b

5. The partial pressure of carbon dioxide is highest in the _____ and lowest in the _____ to allow for passive diffusion of this metabolic waste product.
    a. lung / tissues   b. tissues / lungs
    c. alveolar capillaries / lung   d. pulmonary capillaries / lungs

6.   Diffusion is used to describe the random movement of molecules, such as gas molecules, which tend to move

   a. toward areas containing an equal concentration of particles

   b. from areas of lower concentration to areas of higher concentration

   c. from areas of higher concentration to lower concentration

   d. in a completely random motion

7.   During exercise the PCO_2 in the venous blood returning from a skeletal muscle will be

   a. virtually unchanged

   b. slightly lower than at rest

   c. much lower than at rest

   d. higher than at rest

8.   The length of time a red blood cell remains in the pulmonary and tissue capillaries is generally around

   a. 0.75 seconds at rest and down to 0.3-0.4 seconds during maximal exercise

   b. 0.75 seconds in the pulmonary capillaries and varying in the tissue capillaries between 0.3 and 0.4 seconds

   c. 0.3-0.4 seconds at rest and up to 0.75 seconds during maximal exercise

   d. 0.75 seconds in the tissue capillaries and varying in the pulmonary capillaries between 0.3 and 0.4 seconds

9.   The partial pressure of oxygen at the alveolar level is approximately

   a. 150 mmHg

   b. 100 mmHg

   c. 40 mmHg

   d. 60 mmHg

10.   Diffusion of CO_2 occurs

   a. only during exercise

   b. only during rest

   c. across the visceral pleura

   d. across both the lung and tissue capillary membranes

11.   During exercise the affinity of oxygen for hemoglobin

   a. may be decreased at certain PO_2 levels due to the Bohr effect

   b. remains the same as it is during resting conditions

   c. will be greatly enhanced at all PO_2 levels

   d. may be enhanced at certain PO_2 levels due to the Bohr effect

12. CO_2 is transported in the blood primarily

   a. bound to the heme portion of hemoglobin

   b. bound to the globin portion of hemoglobin

   c. as bicarbonate

   d. dissolved in the plasma

13.   The solubility of carbon dioxide in the plasma is

   a. greater than the solubility of oxygen

   b. very poor

   c. so high that most CO_2 dissolves in the plasma for transport

   d. none of the above

14. Carbon dioxide combines with water to form
   a. carbamino compounds   b. H_2CO_2
   c. carbonic acid   d. none of these answers
15. Removal of carbon dioxide is increased by
   a. hyperventilation   b. hypoventilation
   c. CO_2 rebreathing   d. all of the above
16. The random movement of molecules from areas of high concentration to low concentration
   a. osmosis   b. diffusion
   c. transfusion   d. none of these answers

Key Terms - Define the following terms:

1. Partial pressure

2. Hemoglobin

3. Diffusion

4. Diffusion capacity

5. Hemoconcentration

6. Oxyhemoglobin dissociation curve

7. Bohr Shift

8. Plasma volume

9. Bicarbonate

10. The a-vO_2 difference

Key Concepts - Review your lecture notes and the textbook. You should be able to answer the following questions:

♦ What are the methods of transport for oxygen in the blood?

♦ How is carbon dioxide transported in the blood?

♦ What is the significance of dissolved oxygen and carbon dioxide?

♦ How may partial pressure be calculated for a given gas?

♦ List the factors which influence the diffusion capacity of a gas?

♦ What effect does exercise have on hemoconcentration?

♦ Describe the various types of anemia and their relationship to exercise training.

♦ Which factors cause the Bohr shift?

♦ What is the physiological significance of the Bohr shift?

♦ How is the transport of oxygen influenced by carbon dioxide levels?

Examine the diagrams below. Indicate, in the numbered areas, the mode of CO_2 transport within the blood. Then indicate the percentage of CO_2 transported via each mode.

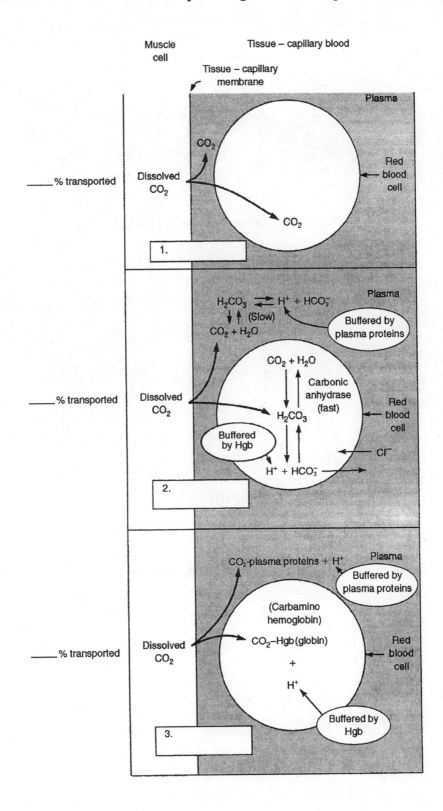

Indicate with an arrow --> or <-- the direction the oxyhemoglobin dissociation curve will shift in response to each parameter listed.

Increased temperature _____   Decreased temperature _____

Increased pH   _____   Decreased pH   _____

Increased PCO_2 _____   Decreased PCO_2 _____

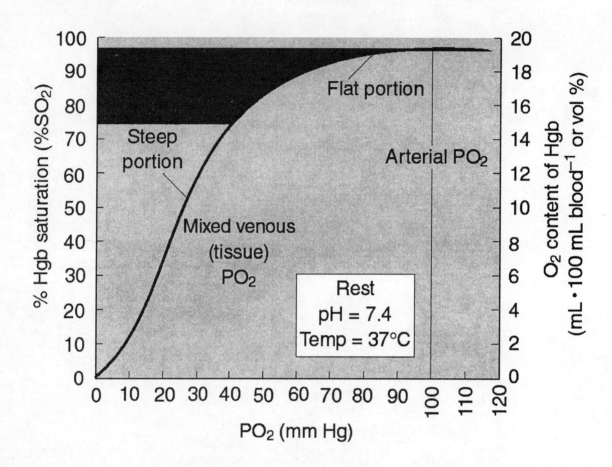

Draw a curve on the above diagram, which would represent exercise conditions.

Post Test

Fill in the blank

1. What does the a-vO_2 difference reveal?_____

2. How does exercise training influence blood plasma volume?_____

3. List the three ways CO_2 is transported in the blood. _____
   _____

4. List the factors which cause the Bohr shift?_____
   _____

5. What effect does exercise training have on hemoconcentration?
   _____

6. The enzyme, _____ located in the red blood cells, drives the reaction combining carbon dioxide and water.

7. The partial pressure of oxygen within the blood is established by the amount of oxygen which is_____.

8. The most important blood protein in regards to buffering H^+ is _____.

9. The level of carbon dioxide in the blood is regulated by making involuntary adjustments in the rate of _____.

10. In addition to carbon dioxide transport, bicarbonate serves as a _____ within the blood.

Multiple Choice - Select the best answer

1. An individual's ability to create a larger a-vO_2 difference after training, might be best explained by
   a. the change in PO_2
   b. breathing in pure O_2
   c. exhaling more CO_2
   d. an increase in the number of mitochondria

2. As oxygen consumption increases we would expect to see
   a. an increase in a-vO_2 difference
   b. a shift to the left of the oxyhemoglobin curve
   c. a decrease in a -vO_2 difference
   d. a downward shift of the oxyhemoglobin curve

3. The reaction between water and CO_2 doesn't occur in the watery plasma because
   a. CO_2 goes by too fast
   b. CO_2 can't bind with plasma water due to its charge
   c. CO_2 dissolves
   d. Carbonic anhydrase is not present

4. The primary buffer in the blood is
   a. oxygen
   b. CO_2
   c. bicarbonate
   d. 2,3 DPG

5. Hyperventilation will
   a. increase PCO_2
   b. increase O_2 levels
   c. decrease PCO_2
   d. decrease PO_2
6. Partial pressure may be calculated by multiplying
   a. total pressure x a-vO_2 difference
   b. total pressure x fractional concentration
   c. gas A x gas B
   d. a-vO_2 difference x fractional concentration
7. Acid base balance is regulated primarily by
   a. the kidneys
   b. the liver
   c. the lungs
   d. both a & c
8. Increasing ventilation rates at sea level will
   a. increase hemoglobin saturation
   b. decrease hemoglobin saturation
   c. not influence hemoglobin saturation
   d. increase RBC number
9. Total oxygen extraction depends upon the oxygen content of the blood and
   a. capillary density
   b. thickness of tissue membranes
   c. PCO_2
   d. all of these answers
10. The amount of oxygen dissolved in the plasma is significant in that it
    a. is the primary transport mode
    b. establishes the PO_2
    c. provides tissues with most of its O_2
    d. determines the rate of glycolysis
11. The red blood cells lack
    a. nuclei
    b. mitochondria
    c. glycolytic capabilities
    d. both a & b
12. Bicarbonate is indirectly derived from the chemical reaction between
    a. CO_2 & H_2CO_3-
    b. O_2 & CO_2
    c. CO_2 & H_2O
    d. CO_2 & HCO_3-

13.	The ratio of the amount of O_2 actually combined with Hgb to the maximal amount which could be combined

a. affinity

b. percent saturation

c. percent dissociation

d. binding ability

14.	The protein portion of hemoglobin actually binds

a. O_2

b. CO_2

c. both O_2 & CO_2

d. neither O_2 or CO_2

15.	The heme portion of the hemoglobin molecule actually binds

a. O_2

b. CO_2

c. both O_2 & CO_2

d. neither O_2 or CO_2

16.	The reduced ability of hemoglobin to bind O_2 when it is saturated with CO_2

a. Bohr effect

b. Boring effect

c. Halogen effect

d. Haldane effect

17.	Training increases the amount of proteins in the blood, this raises the _____ of the blood

a. sodium content

b. osmolality

c. osmosis

d. pH

18.	Oxygen is transported in the blood primarily

a. dissolved in plasma

b. as bicarbonate

c. bound to albumin

d. bound to hemoglobin

19.	CO_2 is transported dissolved in plasma in _____ amounts compared to oxygen

a. the same

b. slightly lower

c. greater

d. drastically lower

20.	The Bohr shift occurs due to (select all correct conditions)

a. increased PCO_2

b. increased temperature

c. increased pH

d. increased 2,3 DPG

21. The oxyhemoglobin dissociation curve illustrates PO_2 levels and its influence on
    a. hemoglobin content
    b. hemoglobin saturation
    c. hemoglobin production
    d. hemoglobin levels

22. The decrease in plasma content of the blood
    a. osmolality
    b. hematocrit
    c. hemoconcentration
    d. hematoma

23. Increased blood temperature may _____hemoglobin saturation with O_2
    a. greatly increase
    b. slightly increase
    c. reduce
    d. prevent

24. The solubility of either oxygen or carbon dioxide will directly influence the amount
    a. dissolved in plasma
    b. bound to hemoglobin
    c. carried as bicarbonate
    d. bound to PO_4

25. CO_2 combines with H_2O to form
    a. bicarbonate
    b. hemoglobin
    c. carbonic acid
    d. citric acid

Answers - Chapter 8

Pretest

1. C
2. C
3. D
4. B
5. B
6. C
7. D
8. A
9. B
10. D
11. A
12. C
13. A
14. C
15. D
16. B

Post Test

Fill in the blank

1. amount of O_2 extracted
2. increased volume
3. bicarbonate, bound to Hgb dissolved in plasma
4. increased temp, PCO_2, 2,3 DPG & decreased pH
5. decreased
6. carbonic anhydrase
7. dissolved in the plasma
8. hemoglobin
9. breathing or respiration
10. buffer

Multiple Choice

1. D
2. A
3. D
4. C
5. C
6. B
7. D
8. C
9. D
10. B
11. D
12. C
13. B
14. B
15. A
16. A
17. B
18. D
19. C
20. A,B,D
21. B
22. C
23. C
24. A
25. C

CHAPTER 9
CARDIOVASCULAR STRUCTURE AND FUNCTION

Lecture Preparation: Multiple Choice

Instructions: After reading the chapter, read each question and the answer choices. Select the choice which BEST answers the question. Check your answers at the back of this chapter, and review any incorrectly answered questions in your textbook.

1. Cardiac Output consists of
   a. heart rate x heart volume
   b. heart volume x respiratory rate
   c. heart rate x stroke volume
   d. heart volume x stroke volume

2. Two factors involved in the redistribution of blood flow during exercise are
   a. vasoconstriction in arterioles in inactive muscles and local factors leading to vasodilation in active muscles
   b. vasoconstriction in arterioles of active muscles and local factors leading to vasodilation in inactive muscles
   c. local factors causing vasoconstriction in arterioles of active muscles and inactive muscles
   d. none of the above

3. The proper sequence of blood traveling through the heart is
   a. right atrium—tricuspid valve—right ventricle—pulmonary valve—pulmonary circulation—left atrium—mitral valve—left ventricle—aortic valve—systemic circulation
   b. right atrium—mitral valve—right ventricle—pulmonary valve—pulmonary circulation—left atrium—tricuspid valve—left ventricle—aortic valve—systemic circulation
   c. right ventricle—mitral valve—right atrium—pulmonary valve—pulmonary circulation—left ventricle—tricuspid valve—left atrium—aortic valve—systemic circulation
   d. left atrium—tricuspid valve—left ventricle—pulmonary valve—pulmonary circulation—right atrium—mitral valve—right ventricle—aortic valve—systemic circulation

4. A difference between the myocardium and skeletal muscle is
   I. cardiac muscle has striations
   II. skeletal muscle uses the sliding filament theory and cardiac muscle does not
   III. cardiac muscle is connected by intercalated disks
   IV. skeletal muscle has mitochondria
   V. cardiac muscle has an inherent rhythm or auto rhythmicity
      a. I, III & V
      b. II & IV
      c. II, III & IV
      d. III & V

5. The proper sequence of blood traveling through the systemic circulation is
   a. arteries—capillaries—arterioles—veins—venules—vena cava
   b. vena cava—venules—capillaries—veins—arterioles—arteries
   c. aorta—arteries—capillaries—arterioles—veins—vena cava
   d. aorta—arteries—arterioles—capillaries—venules—veins—vena cava

6.   Local factors contributing to vasodilation of vascular smooth muscle in skeletal muscle arterioles are

I.   increased CO_2

II.   increased temperature

III. decreased pH

IV. decreased O_2

    a. I & II

    b. I & III

    c. I, II & IV

    d. I, II, III & IV

7.   The pause of the action potential at the atrio ventricular node allows for

a. blood to flow from the atria into the ventricles

b. blood to be released from the ventricles

c. none of the above

d. both a & b

8.   As cardiac output increases with exercise

a. heart rate rises as stroke volume decreases

b. respiratory rate rises before stroke volume

c. heart volume rises as heart rate decreases

d. stroke volume rises as heart rate rises

9.   On an ECG, the beginning of ventricular repolarization is represented by

a. the QRS complex

b. the T wave

c. the S-T segment

d. the P wave

10.   Factors effecting resistance to flow are

I.   the length of the blood vessel

II.   the viscosity of the blood

III. the diameter of the vessel

IV. the vascular smooth muscle tone

    a. I & II

    b. I, II, & III

    c. II, & IV

    d. I, II, III, & IV

11.   The most critical factor affecting resistance to flow is

a. the radius of the blood vessel

b. the length of the blood vessel

c. the blood viscosity

d. all of the above are equally important

12. *Starling's Law of the Heart* pertains to

   a. the mechanism in which an increase in diastolic volume increases stroke volume to meet the demands of exercise

   b. the mechanism in which a change in end diastolic volume produces a change in stroke volume such that the left and right ventricles keep pace with each other

   c. the mechanism in which a decrease in diastolic volume leads to a longer ventricular refilling time

   d. the mechanism in which a decrease in diastolic volume leads to a more forceful ventricular systole

13. *Cardiovascular Drift* refers to

   a. the gradual rise in a subject's heart rate during endurance exercise of long duration, caused by a decrease in myocardial glycogen stores

   b. the gradual decrease in a subject's heart rate during endurance exercise of long duration, caused by a decrease in stroke volume

   c. the gradual rise in a subject's heart rate during endurance exercise of long duration, caused by a decrease in stroke volume

   d. none of the above

Key Terms - Define the following terms:

1. Cardiac output

2. SA Node

3. AV Node

4. Systole

5. Diastole

6. Myocardial ischemia

7. Inotropic

8. Chronotropic

9. Stroke volume

10. Frank Starling mechanism

11. Preload

12. Rate pressure product

13. Mean arterial blood pressure

14. Cardiovascular drift

15. Mitral valve

16. EKG

17. Arrhythmia

Key Concepts - Review your lecture notes and the textbook. You should be able to answer the following questions:

- What is a cardiac cycle?

- What is a heart murmur?

- How does the heart work as a functional syncytium?

- Outline the conduction pathway which carries an action potential across the heart.

- What is the role of the S-A node?

- What factors influence preload?

- What factors influence cardiac output during exercise?

- How is cardiac performance measured?

- What does the ejection fraction indicate?

- How does the skeletal muscle pump contribute to cardiac output?

- How does the cardiac cycle change during exercise?

- What mechanisms are involved in the redistribution of blood flow as one transitions from rest to exercise?

Examine the diagram below, then indicate the range of blood pressure within each of the listed areas.

Left ventricle	_____to_____	
Aorta	_____to_____	
Arteries	_____to_____	
Arterioles	_____to_____	
Capillaries	_____to_____	
Venules	_____to_____	
Veins	_____to_____	
Right atrium	_____to_____	

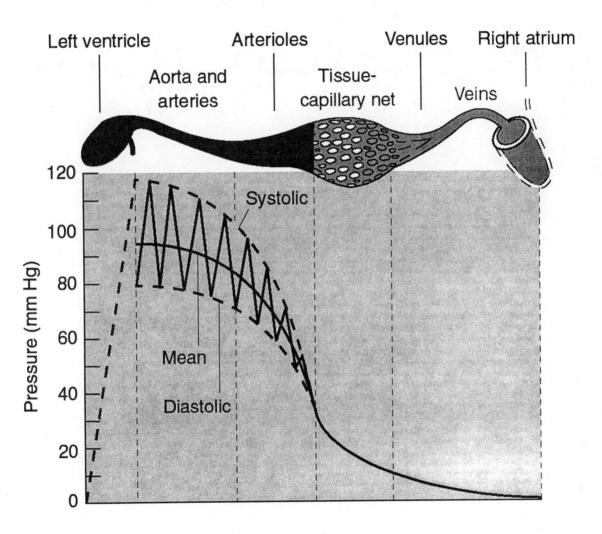

Label the following diagram using the terms provided in the word bank.

Word Bank

P wave	Q wave	R wave	S wave	T wave
QRS complex	S-T segment	P-R interval	R-R interval	isoelectric line

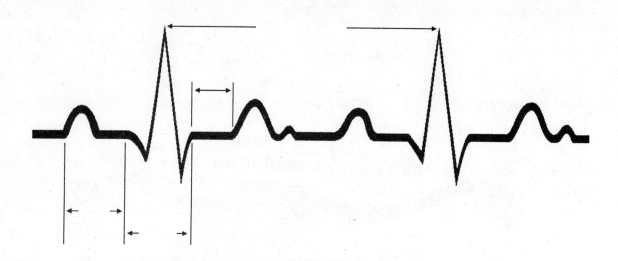

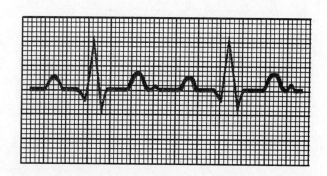

Indicate the mechanical event associated with the following electrical events:

P wave _____

QRS complex _____

S-T segment _____

T wave _____

Label the following diagram using the terms provided in the word bank.

Word Bank

S-A node	A-V node	Bundle of HIS	Right bundle branch
Perkinjie fibers	Right atrium	Left atrium	Left bundle branch
Right ventricle	Left ventricle	Vena cava	Interventricular septum

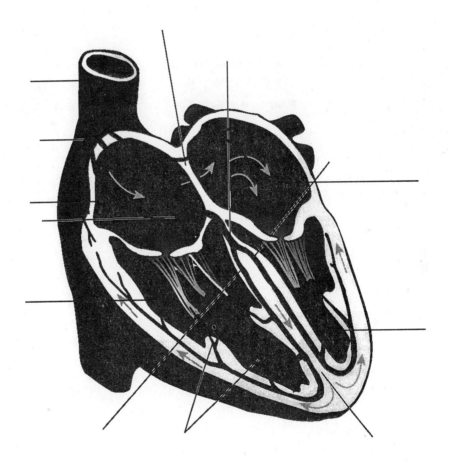

Post Test

Fill in the blank

1. What does a-vO$_2$ difference reveal? _____

2. The volume of blood in the left ventricle just before systole is referred to as _____.

3. The rate pressure product indicates the _____ of the heart.

4. Heart rate times stroke volume is equal to _____.

5. An efficient circulatory system would be indicated by a _____HR coupled with a _____SV.

6. Comparing females to males, one would expect the female's SV to be _____and their HR _____during the same relative submaximal exercise.

7. As heart rate increases during exercise, the time intervals for systole and diastole _____.

8. The vessels supplying inactive tissue respond by _____ during exercise.

9. Local metabolites such as adenosine, CO$_2$, lactate, and nitrous oxide cause _____ in the vessels.

10. The _____ equation is written: cardiac output = VO$_2$ / a-vO$_2$ difference

Multiple Choice

1. The two major components of cardiac performance are
   a. heart rate and blood pressure
   b. heart rate and stroke volume
   c. contractility and distensibility
   d. blood pressure and contractility

2. Factors influencing total peripheral resistance include
   a. viscosity, flow, pressure
   b. pressure, diameter, length of vessel
   c. diameter, length of vessel, flow
   d. diameter, viscosity, length of vessel

3. Which of the following correctly depicts a portion of the blood flow pattern within the heart?
   a. right atria, pulmonary valve, right ventricle, pulmonary artery
   b. left atria, mitral valve, left ventricle, aortic valve
   c. right atria, bicuspid valve, right ventricle, pulmonary valve
   d. left atria, bicuspid valve, left ventricle, pulmonary artery

4. An increase in a-vO$_2$ difference might be explained by
   a. the change in PO$_2$ experienced at altitude (short term)
   b. breathing in pure O$_2$
   c. exhaling more CO$_2$
   d. an increase in the number of mitochondria

5. As exercise intensity increases, preload
   a. increases
   b. decreases slightly
   c. remains the same
   d. decreases drastically

6. An increase in end diastolic volume would influence which of the following most immediately or directly?
   a. blood pressure
   b. stroke volume
   c. contraction time
   d. perfusion

7. As oxygen consumption increases we would expect to see
   a. an increase in a-vO_2 difference   b. a shift to the left of the oxyhemoglobin curve
   c. a decrease in a -vO_2 difference   d. a downward shift of the oxyhemoglobin curve

8. An EKG represents
   a. mechanical heart events   b. electrical events within the heart
   c. rhythm patterns within the heart   d. the heart rate & rhythm

9. On an EKG tracing the P wave represents
   a. ventricular contraction   b. atrial depolarization
   c. atrial repolarization   d. ventricular depolarization

10. Which pattern best describes the SV pattern for an average individual, as exercise intensity increases?
    a. rises then drops to resting levels
    b. rises until about 40% - 60% of VO_2 max, then levels off
    c. rises gradually until max HR is reached
    d. rises rapidly and peaks at lactate threshold

11. Dehydration will cause a reduction in blood volume, the increase in HR needed to compensate creates
    a. maximal HR   b. CV drift
    c. CV flutter   d. HR reserve

12. As exercise intensity increases, we would expect a-vO_2 difference to
    a. decrease   b. remain the same
    c. increase   d. disappear

13. The biggest difference in the cardiac output of an athlete vs. an untrained person is
    a. stroke volume   b. ventricular size
    c. reduced blood pressure   d. increased capillary density

14. From the AV node, the wave of myocardial depolarization passes down the
    a. SA node   b. bundle of HIS
    c. Perkinjie fibers   d. left bundle branch

15. The coronary blood flow is unique in that it experiences a_____ compared to skeletal blood flow
    a. reduced a-vO_2 difference   b. increased a-vO_2 difference
    c. reduced hemoglobin level   d. increased hemoglobin level

16. _____ results when myocardial oxygen demand exceeds supply
    a. murmurs   b. inotropic
    c. ischemia   d. isovolumic filling

17. A term used to describe the state of contractility of the heart
    a. chronotropic   b. inotropic
    c. end diastolic volume   d. afterload

18. Factors which either increase or decrease heart rate
    a. chronotropic   b. inotropic
    c. rate pressure product   d. mean arterial blood pressure

19. An increase in myocardial contractility would cause an increase in the SV at the same EDV. The term used to describe the relationship between SV and a given EDV is
    a. ejection fraction   b. pulse rate
    c. rate pressure product   d. mean arterial blood pressure

20. The volume of blood returned to the right atria via systemic circulation is called
   a. a-vO$_2$ difference   b. pulse rate
   c. ejection fraction   d. venous return

21. The volume of blood returned to the right atria may be increased by all of the following except
   a. skeletal muscle pump   b. venoconstriction
   c. respiratory muscle pump   d. capillary pump

22. The two major hemodynamic factors are
   a. blood pressure & HR   b. blood pressure & resistance
   c. HR & resistance   d. blood pressure & viscosity

23. Systolic blood pressure - diastolic blood pressure =
   a. ejection fraction   b. mean arterial blood pressure
   c. preload   d. pulse pressure

24. The factor which has the greatest influence on peripheral resistance
   a. heart rate   b. vessel diameter
   c. blood viscosity   d. vessel length

25. Chronically elevated blood pressure, with no known cause
   a. labile hypertension   b. exercise induced hypertension
   c. essential hypertension   d. hyperemia

Answers - Chapter 9

Pretest

1. C
2. A
3. A
4. D
5. D
6. D
7. A
8. D
9. B
10. D
11. A
12. B
13. C

Post Test

Fill in the blank

1. oxygen extraction
2. end diastolic volume or preload
3. workload/O$_2$ demand

4. cardiac output

5. lower, larger

6. lower, higher

7. decrease

8. vasoconstricting

9. vasodilation

10. Fick

Multiple Choice

1. B

2. D

3. B

4. D

5. A

6. B

7. A

8. B

9. B

10. B

11. B

12. C

13. A

14. B

15. B

16. C

17. B

18. A

19. A

20. D

21. D

22. B

23. D

24. B

25. C

CHAPTER 10
CARDIORESPIRATORY CONTROL

Lecture Preparation: Multiple Choice

Instructions: After reading the chapter, read each question and the answer choices. Select the choice which BEST answers the question. Check your answers at the back of this chapter, and review any incorrectly answered questions in your textbook.

1. Electrical stimulation of the brain stem from neural and humoral sources elicits change in respiration mainly through

    a. altering rate and depth of pulmonary ventilation

    b. increasing blood flow through the apices of the lungs

    c. directly altering the alveolar ventilation-perfusion ratio

    d. none of the above

2. Electrical stimulation of the brain stem from neural and humoral sources elicits change in circulation mainly through

    a. altering heart rate and stroke volume

    b. vasodilation and vasoconstriction

    c. affecting venous return through venoconstriction

    d. all of the above

3. Decreased heart rate and stroke volume may be indicative of

    I.   increased vagal stimulation

    II.   decreased sympathetic stimulation

    III. decreased vagal stimulation

    IV.   increased sympathetic stimulation

    a. I only

    b. I & II

    c. III only

    d. IV only

4. Receptors facilitating negative feedback to the cardiac control centers in response to a transluminal elastic stretch of the carotid arteries are the carotid

    a. chemoreceptors

    b. mechanoreceptors

    c. stretch receptors

    d. baroreceptors

5. At rest, baroreceptors regulate

    a. pH

    b. PO_2

    c. blood pressure

    d. all of the above

6. In anticipation of exercise
   a. there is an increase in NE released at the SA node and a decrease in acetylcholine
   b. there is an increase in NE released at the SA node and an increase in acetylcholine
   c. there is a decrease in NE released at the SA node and an increase in acetylcholine
   d. neither NE nor acetylcholine are released at the SA node of the heart's conduction pathway

7. Exercise-induced hyperpnea refers to
   a. increase in the rate of breathing
   b. increase in the depth of breathing
   c. regulation of arterial PO_2, PCO_2 and pH
   d. all of the above

8. The respiratory area during exercise is under the influence of
   a. descending impulses of the brain's motor regions and cerebral chemoreceptors sensitive to H^+
   b. ascending impulses from the lung and airway receptors, peripheral chemoreceptors and lung CO_2 receptors
   c. ascending impulses from intercostal and diaphragm muscle receptors and ergoreceptors of active skeletal muscles
   d. all of the above

Key Terms - Define the following terms:

1. Ventilation
2. Medulla Oblongata
3. Mechanoreceptors
4. Metaboreceptors
5. Baroreceptors
6. Autonomic nervous system
7. Sympathetic nervous system
8. Parasympathetic nervous system
9. Catecholamines
10. Hyperpnea
11. Central comand

Key Concepts - Review your lecture notes and the textbook. You should be able to answer the following questions:

- What is the role of the medulla oblongata in controlling ventilatory rate and depth?

- Describe the function of the parasympathetic nervous system in regards to controlling cardiorespiratory processes.

- What is the role of the sympathetic nervous system in controlling cardiorespiratory responses?

- Why do heart rate and ventilation increase prior to beginning a bout of exercise?

- Describe the various local metabolites and the effect they have on the cardiorespiratory response?

- How is blood pressure regulated during exercise?

- Where are the peripheral chemoreceptors located?

- Where are the baroreceptors located?

- How do chemoreceptors and baroreceptors regulate one's cardiorespiratory response?

- Compare and contrast metaboreceptors and mechanoreceptors.

Examine the diagram below. For each receptor listed, indicate the area where it would be located and the stimuli to which it responds.

Receptors	Area	Stimuli		Stimuli – Word Bank
Mechanoreceptors	____	_____	PO_2	Temperature
Baroreceptors	____	_____	PCO_2	Pressure
Metaboreceptors	____	_____	H^+	Mechanical movement
Medulla oblongata	____	_____	pH	

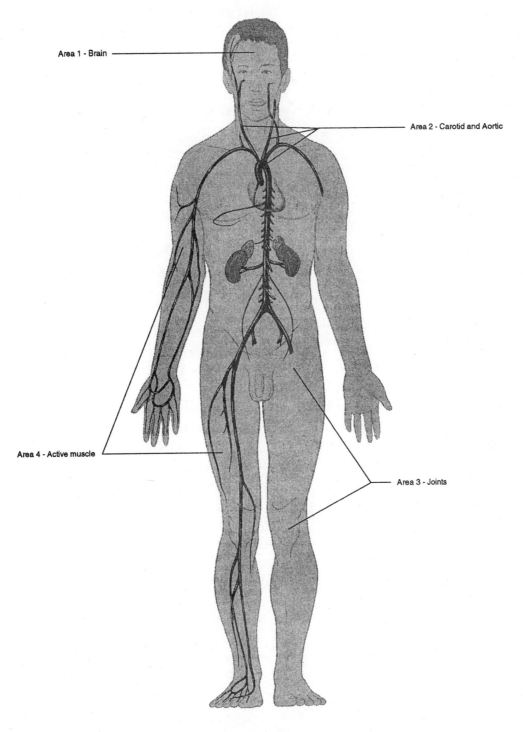

Area 1 - Brain

Area 2 - Carotid and Aortic

Area 4 - Active muscle

Area 3 - Joints

Post Test

Fill in the blank

1. Systolic blood pressure should _____ in response to exercise.

2. The _____ nerves cause an increase in heart rate.

3. Diastolic blood pressure should _____ or _____ in response to exercise.

4. The central processing of cardiorespiratory control occurs predominantly in the _____.

5. Changes in blood or cerebral spinal fluid chemical properties are classified as _____ stimuli.

6. The _____ receptors are primarily sensitive to pressure.

7. The _____ receptors are primarily responsive to metabolic changes or metabolic by products.

8. Nerves innervating the heart and blood vessels belong to the _____ nervous system.

9. Nerves which release norepinephrine are classified as _____ nerves.

10. Cholinergic nerves release the neurotransmitter, _____.

Multiple Choice

1. The vagus nerves evoke the following response from the heart
   a. arrhythmias
   b. tachycardia
   c. decreased rate
   d. increased rate

2. During exercise, increases in heart rate above 100 BPM are primarily due to
   a. vagal stimulation
   b. increased sympathetic tone
   c. vagal withdrawal
   c. sympathetic withdrawal

3. The accumulation of local metabolites such as adenosine, lactate, and nitrous oxide causes
   a. vasodilation
   b. vasoconstriction
   c. diversion of blood flow
   d. pooling of blood

4. Beta blockers are primarily responsible for
   a. enhancing catecholamine response
   b. enhancing acetylcholine
   c. blunting catecholamine response
   d. blunting acetylcholine

5. The baroreceptors are most sensitive to _____ changes
   a. joint pressure
   b. atrial chamber size
   c. ventricular wall
   d. transluminal stretch

6. Chemoreceptors are sensitive to a reduction in _____
   a. PO_2
   b. PCO_2
   c. hydrogen ions
   d. potassium ions

7. Anticipation of exercise may increase heart rate via
   a. sympathetic stimuli
   b. sympathetic inhibition
   c. parasympathetic stimuli
   d. parasympathetic inhibition

8. The increase in blood pressure during static exercise, is directly related to
   a. exercise duration
   b. exercise frequency
   c. intensity of exercise
   d. relative intensity & amount of muscle mass involved

9. The increase in blood pressure during dynamic exercise is directly related to the
   a. mode
   b. intensity of exercise
   c. frequency
   d. duration

10. At near maximal efforts, the parasympathetic activity is
    a. very apparent
    b. decreased slightly
    c. dominant
    d. almost nonexistent

11. The rapid rise in ventilation occurring during the initiation of exercise is primarily due to
    a. negative feedback from tissues
    b. feedforward control
    c. peripherally dictated
    d. lactate build up

12. An increase in ventilatory rate may be referred to as exercise
    a. hypercapnia
    b. hypertrophy
    c. hyperpnea
    d. hyperplasia

13. Increases in the rate and depth of breathing are due to increased stimulation of the
    a. diaphragm
    b. lungs
    c. external obliques
    d. internal obliques

14. Mechanical movements are detected by the
    a. mechanoreceptors
    b. barorecptors
    c. metaboreceptors
    d. pressoceptors

15. Resting bradycardia, resulting from exercise training, is due to
    a. decreased sympathetic activity
    b. increased sympathetic activity
    c. decreased parasympathetic activity
    d. increased parasympathetic activity

Answers - Chapter 10

Pretest

1. A
2. D
3. B
4. D
5. C
6. A
7. A
8. D

Post Test

Fill in the blank

1. increase
2. cardiac accelerator
3. remain the same / slightly increase
4. Medulla oblongata
5. humoral
6. baro or mechanoreceptors
7. metaboreceptors
8. autonomic
9. adrenergic
10. acetylcholine

Mutiple Choice

1. C
2. B
3. A
4. C
5. D
6. A
7. D
8. D
9. B
10. D
11. B
12. C
13. A
14. A
15. D

CHAPTER 11
METHODS FOR ANAEROBIC TRAINING AND PHYSIOLOGIC RESPONSE

Lecture Preparation: Multiple Choice

Instructions: After reading the chapter, read each question and the answer choices. Select the choice which BEST answers the question. Check your answers at the back of this chapter, and review any incorrectly answered questions in your textbook.

1. Intermittent exercise relies greater on the lactic acid system when the relief period consists of
   a. low intensity exercise or work relief period between repetitions of an interval
   b. complete rest without exercise between repetitions of an interval
   c. a very long relief period, such as with a work-relief ratio of 1:3
   d. none of the above

2. Sprint training should include
   a. at least 6 seconds of sprinting and long recovery intervals
   b. at least 15 seconds of sprinting and short recovery intervals
   c. no more than 45 seconds of sprinting with work-relief ratio of 3:1
   d. at least 6 seconds of sprinting with a work-relief ratio of 1:1

3. Cycling one's training regimen in an effort to peak prior to competitions
   a. circuit training
   b. periodization
   c. cross training
   d. plyometric training

4. Utilizing a prestretch followed by quick explosive concentric contractions
   a. circuit training
   b. periodization
   c. cross training
   d. plyometric training

5. Anaerobic training depends to a great extent upon
   a. the Krebs cycle
   b. beta oxidation
   c. glycoysis & the ATP-CP system
   d. aerobic glycoysis

6. Progressing through a series of exercises designed to compliment one another and form a complete training session.
   a. circuit training
   b. periodization
   c. cross training
   d. plyometric training

7. Anaerobic athletes should train at a heart rate which
   a. is above lactate threshold
   b. can be maintained for 60 minutes
   c. can be maintained for 30 minutes
   d. can be maintained for 90 minutes

8. Off-season training for anaerobic athletes should consist of
   a. high intensity runs
   b. low intensity aerobic work, weight lifting
   c. weight lifting only
   d. total rest

9. Repeated bouts of high intensity work alternated with recovery periods
   a. periodization
   b. cycling training
   c. interval training
   d. continuous training

10. Anaerobic adaptations within skeletal muscle show a preferential
    a. atrophy of Type I fibers
    b. hypertrophy of Type I fibers
    c. atrophy of Type II fibers
    d. hypertrophy of Type II fibers

Key Terms - Define the following terms:

1. Overload Principle
2. Specificity
3. Interval training
4. Frequency
5. Intensity
6. Duration
7. Periodization
8. Training effect
9. Detraining
10. Progression
11. Recovery
12. Mode
13. Work interval
14. Relief interval

Key Concepts - Review your lecture notes and the textbook. You should be able to answer the following questions:

- ◆ Describe the various ways which overload may be achieved.

- ◆ Describe the physiological basis for specificity.

- ◆ What does interval training involve?

- ◆ Why is it important to warm up and cool down?

- ◆ How might a coach identify the predominant energy system utilized for a specific activity?

- ◆ How can the proper work intensities and relief intervals be determined?

- ◆ What types of training activities should be utilized during the off-season, pre-season, and in-season?

- ◆ Describe what occurs during periods of detraining.

- ◆ What physiological changes occur in response to anaerobic training?

Post Test

Multiple Choice

1. The energy sources for a given activity depends upon
    a. time & frequency   b. time & intensity
    c. time only   d. frequency only

2. Overload may be achieved by increasing
    a. intensity   b. frequency
    c. duration   d. all of these answers

3. Overload should be obtained
    a. immediately   b. only in-season
    c. progressively   d. only in pre-season

4. The recommended training frequency for anaerobic improvement is _____ times a week.
    a. 2   b. 3–4
    c. 5–6   d. 7

5. The number of training sessions per day for anaerobic events
    a. 1–2   b. 3
    c. 4   d. 5

6. Athletes should spend most training time performing their specific sport with a high intensity during
    a. off-season   b. pre-season
    c. in-season   d. all phases

7. Athletes should spend most of their time on sport specific skill development & maintenance conditioning during
    a. off-season   b. pre-season
    c. in-season   d. all phases

8. The structured sequential development of physiologic capacity accomplished by blocking training times
    a. interval training   b. Fartlek training
    c. periodization   d. cyclic training

9. The physiological reasons for performing a warm-up do NOT include increasing

    a. body temperature   b. blood flow

    c. reaction time   d. enzyme activity

10. Stretching exercises should be

    a. preceded by a general low intensity, sport specific activity

    b. ballistic in nature

    c. the very first thing an athlete should do

    d. the major focus of every workout session

11. One important reason to perform a cool down is to help remove

    a. PO_4^- b. O_2

    c. HCO_3^- d. lactic acid

12. The relief interval usually includes all of the following except

    a. walking   b. light jogging

    c. moderate exercise   d. sitting still

13. One of the major benefits of interval training involves a(n) _____ of the actual work performed.

    a. increased volume   b. increased intensity

    c. decreased intensity   d. decreased volume

14. Anaerobic training programs can be guided by all of the following except

    a. pace   b. heart rate

    c. partner pacing   d. lactate threshold

15. Adaptations to anaerobic training include all of the following except

    a. increased glycolytic enzyme activity

    b. increased ATP stores

    c. increased triglyceride stores

    d. increased PC stores

Answers - Chapter 11

Pretest

1. A
2. C
3. B
4. D
5. C
6. A
7. A
8. B
9. C
10. D

Post Test

1. B
2. D
3. C
4. B
5. A
6. B
7. C
8. C
9. C
10. A
11. D
12. D
13. B
14. C
15. C

CHAPTER 12
METHODS FOR AEROBIC TRAINING AND PHYSIOLOGIC RESPONSE

Lecture Preparation: Multiple Choice

Instructions: After reading the chapter, read each question and the answer choices. Select the choice which BEST answers the question. Check your answers at the back of this chapter, and review any incorrectly answered questions in your textbook.

1.   The performance time for an activity can be used to establish

a. the overload principle for that activity

b. the primary energy system for that activity

c. the quality of the performance for all activities

d. all of the above

2.   Training intensity can be identified from

I.   heart rate response to the exercise

II.   lactate threshold and ventilatory effort

III. core temperature and sweating

IV. exercise mode

a. I only

b. I & II

c. I, II & IV

d. I, II, III & IV

3.   The fundamental step in formulating a training program is

a. to identify the specific energy system for the activity and train that system according to the overload principle

b. to make sure all the energy systems are being trained equally to allow for proper balance and improved performance

c. to always train at a higher intensity and duration than what the activity or sport itself entails

d. to always train at a lower intensity and duration than what the activity or sport itself entails to prevent injury

4.   Overload may include

I.   amount of weight lifted

II.   intensity

III. frequency

IV. duration

a. I only

b. I &III

c. II, III & IV

d. I, II, III & IV

5. Both training at 80% of their aerobic capacity, a detrained individual and an endurance athlete should have

    a. very different heart rates, with the endurance athlete's heart rate being lower

    b. very different heart rates, with the detrained individual's heart rate being lower

    c. similar heart rates

    d. similar rates of lactic acid production

6. One of the best methods for establishing proper exercise intensity is to determine

    a. maximal heart rate

    b. resting heart rate

    c. target heart rate

    d. none of these answers

7. Heart rate reserve (HRR) is

    a. ventricular contractions remaining at the end of cardiac drift

    b. 220 - your age

    c. 220 - your resting heart rate (RHR)

    d. your resting heart rate (RHR) subtracted from your maximum heart rate (HRmax)

8. A few good recommendations for an off season training program would be

    I.   running at a high intensity every day

    II. partaking in competitive performances on a regular basis

    III. engage in a form of cross training (different sports than the athlete's main sport)

    IV. weight training 3 days per week to maintain strength

        a. I & II

        b. I, III & IV

        c. I, II, III & IV

        d. III & IV

9. The purpose of a warm down is

    a. to prevent the pooling of blood in the extremities exercised by allowing the muscle pump to facilitate venous return.

    b. To decrease muscle lactic acid levels more rapidly and enhance recovery from fatigue.

    c. To decrease blood lactic acid levels more rapidly and enhance recovery from fatigue.

    d. all of the above.

10. A few good recommendations for an off season training program would be

    I.   running at a high intensity 3 days per week for 8 weeks.

    II. partaking in competitive performances on a regular basis.

    III. engage in a form of cross training (different sports rather than the athlete's main sport).

    IV. Weight training 3 days per week for 8 weeks.

        a. I & II

        b. I, III & IV

        c. III & IV

        d. I, II, III & IV

11. A person's maximum heart rate (HRmax) can be approximated by

    a. subtracting their RHR from 220

    b. subtracting their age from 220

    c. adding their age to their HRR

    d. all of the above are accepted methods

12. An effective intensity at which an endurance athlete should train to seek the most benefit is
    a. at or slightly below anaerobic threshold
    b. at or slightly above anaerobic threshold
    c. at 60% of HRmax
    d. at 95% of HRR

13. Long distance workouts performed at one's spontaneous pace
    a. cross training
    b. circuit training
    c. tempo training
    d. Fartlek

14. Endurance exercise training is based upon
    a. low to moderate intensity exercise with relief periods between bouts
    b. complete rest without exercise between repetitions of very intense intervals
    c. a very long relief period, with very short work intervals
    d. none of the above

15. Endurance training should include
    a. periods of recovery
    b. dietary supplements
    c. sprint training every third day
    d. a very high protein diet

16. Long slow distance running for most runners should
    a. cover approximately 2 to 5 times the distance of their event
    b. be performed at 70–75% of the athlete's HRR
    c. be performed at 85% of the athlete's HRmax
    d. all of the above

Key Terms - Define the following terms:

1. Cross training

2. Tempo training

3. Fartlek training

4. Detraining

5. Retraining

6. Overtraining

7. Tapering

Key Concepts - Review your lecture notes and the textbook. You should be able to answer the following questions:

- ◆ How can heart rate be utilized as a guide for establishing training intensity?

- ◆ What does Fartlek training involve?

- ◆ How is tempo training different than interval sprinting?

- ◆ What are the physiological advantages of cross training?

- ◆ Describe the changes which occur within skeletal muscle as a result of aerobic training.

- ◆ Describe the structural and functional changes, observable at rest, during submaximal and maximal exercise, which occur as a result of aerobic training.

- ◆ How does heredity influence one's ability to benefit from training?

- ◆ What are the major signs and symptoms of overtraining?

- ◆ Describe the general outcome resulting from periods of detraining.

- ◆ Describe the training effects which are responsible for an increased ability to perform aerobic exercise.

Post Test

Multiple Choice

1. During aerobic exercise, the predominant muscle fiber recruited is Type
    a. I   b. IIa
    c. IIb   d. IIc

2. Progressive overload involves the manipulation of all the following variables except
    a. intensity   b. frequency
    c. mode   d. duration

3. To induce aerobic training adaptations, exercise intensity should be performed at least between
    a. 30–50% VO_2max   b. 30–50% max heart rate
    c. 50–85% VO_2max   d. 95–100% max heart rate

4. Two heart rate based methods for determining training intensity are
    a. reservation method   b. heart rate reserve
    c. max minus age   d. percentage of maximum

5. The recommended training frequency for most athletic events is _____ times per week
    a. 1–2   b. 4–6
    c. 7   d. 2–3

6. Decreasing training duration prior to an event is known as
    a. Fartlek   b. pacing
    c. tempo   d. tapering

7. The best method for recovering from aerobic exercise, when another bout is to be performed within one hour, is to
    a. lie down   b. sit down
    c. alternate sitting & lying   d. exercise moderately

8. Training of moderate duration and high intensity is called _____ training
    a. Fartlek   b. tempo
    c. taper   d. interval

9. An exercise training system in which relief and work intervals are not precisely timed is called
a. Fartlek   b. tempo
c. taper   d. interval

10. The type of training which involves the transfer of effects gained from one mode to another is called ___ training
a. Fartlek   b. tempo
c. cross   d. interval

11. Skeletal muscle changes in response to exercise training all lead to improved ability to
a. transport FFA   b. generate ATP
c. transport glucose   d. synthesize protein

12. Skeletal muscles experience an increased capacity to oxidize glycogen into H_2O and CO_2. Subcellular adaptations responsible for this improved oxidizing capability include an increase in all of the following except
a. number of mitochondria   b. size of mitochondria
c. oxidative enzymes   d. saturation of hemoglobin

13. During heavy but submaximal exercise greater fat oxidation accounts for which of the following
a. glycogen sparing   b. total fat depletion
c. PC depletion   d. protein depletion

14. Aerobic exercise training results in a(n) _____ ability to interconvert Type I and II muscle fiber types
a. slightly increased   b. decreased
c. non altered   d. significantly increased

15. Aerobic training adaptations which are apparent at rest include all of the following except
a. decreased heart rate   b. increased blood volume
c. increased capillary density   d. decreased stroke volume

16. The cardiac hypertrophy experienced by endurance athletes is usually characterized by increased
a. ventricular wall thickness   b. atrial wall thickness
c. ventricular chamber size   d. atrial chamber size

17. The cardiac hypertrophy experienced by non-endurance athletes is usually characterized by increased
a. ventricular wall thickness   b. atrial wall thickness
c. ventricular chamber size   d. atrial chamber size

18. The reduction in resting heart rate resulting from a training program is predominantly due to
a. increased sympathetic tone   b. increased parasympathetic tone
c. decreased autonomic tone   d. decreased parasympathetic tone

19. The delivery of oxygen to the tissues is greatly enhanced by an increase in which of the following?
a. mitochondrial number   b. oxidative enzymes
c. glycolytic enzymes   d. capillary density

20. Trained individuals experience a(n) _____ in oxygen consumption during submaximal exercise, when compared to rest.
a. increase   b. decrease
c. no change   d. either b or c

21. Trained individuals experience an increased a-vO_2 difference which helps explain the _____ in muscle blood flow per kilogram of active muscle during submaximal work loads.
a. increase   b. decrease
c. unaltered   d. either a or c

22.	With the exception of elite athletes, _____ is not a limiting factor for max VO$_2$.
	a. pulmonary function			b. hemoglobin levels
	c. cardiac output			d. stroke volume

23.	Bone density increases with the deposition of _____ in the bone matrix
	a. sodium phosphate			b. calcium phosphate
	c. sodium caltrate			d. pure calcium

24.	Reduced training frequencies _____ maintain training adaptations for several months.
	a. can not				b. can
	c. usually fail to			d. absolutely fail to

25.	Previous aerobic training _____ retraining
	a. speeds up the effects of		b. slows down the effects of
	c. has no effect on			d. allows one to achieve higher fitness levels with

Answers - Chapter 12

Pretest

1.	B
2.	B
3.	A
4.	D
5.	C
6.	C
7.	D
8.	D
9.	D
10.	B
11.	B
12.	A
13.	D
14.	A
15.	A
16.	D

Post Test

1. A
2. C
3. B
4. B, D
5. B
6. D
7. D
8. B
9. A
10. C
11. B
12. D
13. A
14. C
15. D
16. C
17. A
18. B
19. D
20. A
21. B
22. A
23. B
24. B
25. C

CHAPTER 13
DEVELOPMENT OF MUSCULAR STRENGTH, ENDURANCE AND FLEXIBILITY

Lecture Preparation: Multiple Choice

Instructions: After reading the chapter, read each question and the answer choices. Select the choice which BEST answers the question. Check your answers at the back of this chapter, and review any incorrectly answered questions in your textbook.

1.   The physiological principle in which strength and endurance are developed is called

   a. specificity of training

   b. training mode

   c. overload

   d. intensity

2.   When a muscle shortens while lifting a constant load, the tension developed depends on

   a. the speed of the shortening

   b. the angle of pull

   c. the length of the muscle

   d. all of the above

3.   The law of specificity is applied to improve the strength or endurance of a certain skill if

   I.   the program includes exercises for the muscle groups the skill involves

   II.   the program includes sufficient cross training for recovery

   III. the program includes exercises that simulate the motor patterns the skill involves

   IV. the program is performed with a specific frequency

      a. I & III only

      b. I & IV only

      c. I , III & IV only

      d. I, II, III & IV

4.   Flexibility is

   a. related to health

   b. possibly related to athletic performance

   c. the range of motion in a joint

   d. all of the above

5.   At 60% of its resting length, the tension a muscle develops is near zero because

   a. the actin filaments are pulled completely out of the range of the cross-bridges

   b. there is an overlap of actin filaments so that the filament from one side interferes with the coupling potential of the other side

   c. the angle of pull is such that optimum tension is reduced

   d. all of the above

6. Isotonic contractions using constant loads are at a disadvantage because

   a. the heaviest weight that can be lifted is the weight that can be lifted at the weakest angle of pull on the muscle only

   b. at certain joint angles the muscle will not be exerting tension near its maximal force

   c. maximum tension can not be distributed completely through the range of motion

   d. all of the above

7. When tension is developed without a change in external length of the muscle, _____ is being performed

   a. an isokinetic contraction

   b. an eccentric contraction

   c. a concentric contraction

   d. an isometric contraction

8. Hypertrophy of muscle fibers can be attributed to

   I.   increased number and size of myofibrils per muscle fiber

   II. increased capillary density per muscle fiber

   III. increased total amount of contractile protein, particularly the myosin filament

   IV. increased amount and strength of connective tissues

       a. I only

       b. I & III only

       c. I, II & III only

       d. I, II, III & IV

9. Skeletal muscle changes that have been proven to occur in response to resistance training programs are

   a. interconversion of fast-twitch and slow-twitch fibers and decrease in Type II:Type I fiber area

   b. increases in concentrations of creatine, PC, ATP and glycogen within the muscle

   c. an increase in mitochondria density and ATP turnover enzyme activities (e.g. myokinase)

   d. all of the above

10. The following is true concerning delayed muscular soreness

   I.   it is pain that develops 24 to 48 hours following a bout of exercise

   II. it is most pronounced following eccentric muscular contractions

   III. it is most likely due to damaged connective tissues

   IV. stretching, proper progression, and vitamin C intake have all been suggested to possibly reduce the likelihood and/or severity of muscular soreness

       a. I & III only

       b. II and III only

       c. I, II & III only

       d. I, II, III & IV

11. The Valsalva maneuver is

   a. attempted expiration against a closed glottis (opening between the vocal cords)

   b. dangerous, as it causes a rise in intrathoracic pressures resulting in a rise in blood pressure

   c. common with isometric contractions

   d. all of the above

12. The resistance training proven to be most effective in comparative studies for improving strength and muscular endurance is

    a. isokinetic programs   b. isometric programs

    c. isotonic programs   d. eccentric programs

13. The one rep max is useful in determining

    a. the number of sets to perform

    b. how many times a week to lift weights

    c. the amount of weight to be lifted by a specific muscle group

    d. none of the above

14. Stretching exercises will improve flexibility or

    a. muscular endurance

    b. recruitment of facilitated motor neurons

    c. explosive muscular power

    d. range of motion

15. A type of stretching exercise which is contraindicated

    a. plyometric training

    b. ballistic

    c. static

    d. proprioceptive neuromuscular facilitation

Key Terms - Define the following terms:

1. Concentric contraction

2. Eccentric contraction

3. Isometric contraction

4. Isokinetic contraction

5. Plyometrics

6. Circuit training

7. One rep max

8. Muscular strength

9. Muscular endurance

10. Flexibility

11. ROM

12. Ballistic stretching

13. Static stretching

14. Torn tissue theory

15. Spasm theory

16. Connective tissue theory

Key Concepts - Review your lecture notes and the textbook. You should be able to answer the following questions:

- ◆ Describe the four basic types of muscular contractions and give an example of each of them.

- ◆ Discuss the differences between muscular strength and endurance.

- ◆ How can an individual determine their one rep max?

- ◆ Describe a basic training program based upon isokinetic contractions.

- ◆ When would an isokinetic program be most useful?

- ◆ How do the training principles apply to strength training programs?

- ◆ Discuss the structural factors which limit an individual's flexibility.

- ◆ Describe the procedures used in performing plyometric training drills.

- ◆ Describe the manner in which a circuit training session might be set up.

- ◆ What are the benefits of establishing a flexibility portion for each of an athlete's workout sessions?

- ◆ Describe the difference between the terms isokinetic and isotonic.

- ◆ Describe the proper manner for incorporating stretching into a workout session.

Indicate which exercises would stretch each muscle or muscle group listed.

Erector spinae	_____	Triceps	_____	Biceps	_____
Gastrocnemius	_____	Soleus	_____	Iliopsoas	_____
Pectoralis major	_____	Deltoids	_____	Trapezius	_____
Rectus abdominus	_____	Quadriceps	_____	Gluteus max	_____

1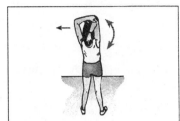

6

2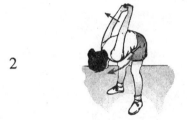

7

3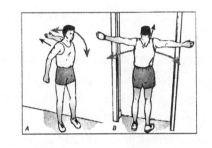

8

4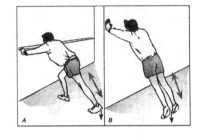

9

5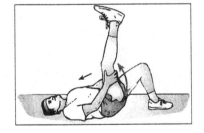

10

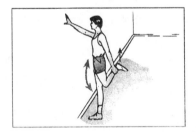

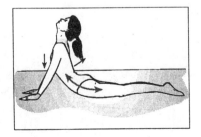

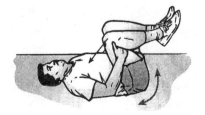

Post Test

Fill in the blank

1. The amount of force a muscle or muscle group can exert maximally in one effort is called_____.

2. The maximal amount of weight a specific muscle group can successfully lift one time only is known as the _____.

3. The strength and _____ of a contraction are important in power movements.

4. Iosmetric contractions measured with a dynamometer represent _____ tests.

5. The ability of a muscle or muscle group to sustain contractions for a period of time is referred to as _____.

6. The resting levels of testosterone have been found to _____ in response to weight training.

7. The increases in isotonic strength per cross sectional area are highly correlated with the percent distribution of _____ fibers.

8. The type of training program in which athletes rotate between a series of stations in a set amount of time is called _____ training.

9. The type of training which attempts to utilize a prestretch to increase stored energy and increase recruitment of facilitated motor neurons is called _____.

10. The range of motion about a joint is defined as _____.

Multiple Choice

1. The type of muscular contraction in which the muscle lengthens despite developing tension
   a. isometric
   b. isokinetic
   c. concentric
   d. eccentric

2. The type of muscular contraction in which the speed is constant throughout the range of motion
   a. isometric
   b. isokinetic
   c. concentric
   d. eccentric

3. Lack of blood flow to a muscle, or ischemia, is the primary cause of
   a. delayed muscle soreness
   b. pain in one's joints
   c. acute muscle soreness
   d. both a & b

4. The amount of tension developed by an intact muscle when it shortens is influenced by all of the following except
   a. parasympathetic tone
   b. initial muscle length
   c. angle of pull on the bone
   d. speed of shortening

5. Equipment which are truly isokinetic accomplish this through a process known as
   a. variable resistance
   b. accommodating resistance
   c. constant resistance
   d. none of these answers

6. The strength of an individual muscle depends upon all of the following except
   a. cross sectional area
   b. connective tissue subcomponents
   c. fiber type composition
   d. overall length of the muscle

102

7. The improvements made during the earliest phase of strength training are probably due to changes or improvements in the
    a. fiber type distribution   b. fat deposition
    c. CNS motor pattern   d. connective tissue

8. The increased size, or hypertrophy, of a muscle is primarily due to the
    a. increase in contractile proteins   b. increased number of myofibrils per fiber
    c. increased size of myofibrils in fibers   d. all of these answers

9. An increase in capillary density is most closely related to an improvement in
    a. strength   b. endurance
    c. flexibility   d. power

10. The splitting of muscle fibers to yield a greater number of fibers is known as
    a. hyperplasia   b. hypertrophy
    c. atrophy   d. fiberlysis

11. Strength training induces all of the following changes except
    a. increases in PC, ATP, & glycogen   b. slight increases in PFK & LDH
    c. interconversion of Type I & II fibers   d. slight decrease in the volume of mitochondria

12. The most probable stimulus for strength and endurance gains include all of the following except
    a. hypoxia   b. frequent high stress
    c. fatigue   d. increased protein consumption

13. The ability of individuals in extreme emergency situations to lift an enormous weight has led to the theoretical explanation that strength is normally inhibited by one's
    a. attitude   b. nervous system
    c. endocrine system   d. muscle fiber types

14. Benefits of weight training include all of the following except
    a. increased testosterone levels at rest   b. increased lean mass
    c. decreased fat mass   d. increased strength

15. The term progressive-resistance exercise has been suggested as a replacement for the term
    a. specificity   b. overload
    c. reversibility   d. recovery

16. The transfer of training from one region of the body to another has _____ at this time.
    a. little support   b. rapidly growing support
    c. been absolutely disproved   d. been put into wide use

17. Pain receptors within the muscle may be stimulated by
    a. lactic acid   b. potassium
    c. calcium   d. both a & b

18. Delayed muscle soreness is greatest following _____ type of muscular contractions.
    a. isometric   b. isokinetic
    c. concentric   d. eccentric

19. Damage to connective tissue is indicated by elevated levels of
    a. hydroxyproline   b. hydroxyvaline
    c. lactic acid   d. bicarbonate

20. Stretching has been shown to be beneficial for
    a. increasing one's ROM   b. preventing soreness
    c. relieving soreness   d. all of these answers

21. The Valsalva maneuver involves changes in
    a. blood pressure   b. capillary density
    c. lactic acid   d. pH of the blood

22. Athletic strength training programs should incorporate movements at speeds _____ those used during actual performance.
    a. slower than   b. approximating
    c. faster than   d. b or c

23. It is generally agreed that strength and endurance once developed, subside at a _____ rate compared to that at which they were developed
    a. faster   b. slower
    c. similar   d. unchanged

24. Sarcopenia is a term used to describe
    a. muscle wasting   b. sore muscles
    c. muscular hypertrophy   d. fiber splitting

25. Performing a stretch, followed by a static contraction against a resistance, then restretching is
    a. proprioceptor neural fusion   b. ballistic neural fusion
    c. static facilitation   d. proprioceptive neuromuscular facilitation

Answers - Chapter 13

Pretest

1. C
2. D
3. A
4. D
5. B
6. D
7. D
8. B
9. B
10. D
11. D
12. D
13. C
14. D
15. B

Post Test

Fill in the blank

1. strength
2. 1 RM

104

3. speed

4. static

5. endurance

6. remain stable

7. Type II

8. circuit

9. plyometrics

10. static flexibility

Multiple Choice

1. D

2. B

3. C

4. A

5. B

6. B

7. C

8. D

9. B

10. A

11. C

12. D

13. B

14. A

15. B

16. A

17. D

18. D

19. A

20. D

21. A

22. D

23. B

24. A

25. D

CHAPTER 14
PHYSICAL ACTIVITY AND HEALTH

Lecture Preparation: Multiple Choice

Instructions: After reading the chapter, read each question and the answer choices. Select the choice which BEST answers the question. Check your answers at the back of this chapter, and review any incorrectly answered questions in your textbook.

1.   Restricted blood flow to the brain tissue

   a. may be the result of a blood clot

   b. may be the result of a cerebral hemorrhage or an aneurysm

   c. is classified as a stroke

   d. all of the above

2.   Exercise may improve lipid profiles by

   a. lowering HDL cholesterol

   b. increasing LDL cholesterol

   c. increasing plasma FFA

   d. increasing HDL cholesterol

3.   People with a systolic blood pressure over 150 mm Hg

   a. have twice the risk of coronary heart disease than the norm

   b. have higher LDL than the norm

   c. have lower HDL than the norm

   d. all of the above

4.   Physical activity may reduce the risk of coronary heart disease by

   I.   lowering blood pressure

   II.   improving glucose tolerance

   III.   decreasing growth hormone production

   IV.   improving myocardial efficiency

       a. I only

       b. I, II & IV

       c. I, III & IV

       d. I, II, III & IV

5.   Risk factors of coronary heart disease which are considered the most important are

   a. cigarette smoking, hypertension and high cholesterol

   b. stress, cigarette smoking and lack of exercise

   c. hypertension, stress and high cholesterol

   d. high cholesterol, lack of exercise, hypertension, and smoking cigarettes

6.   To develop and maintain cardio-respiratory fitness, the American College of Sports Medicine recommends aerobic exercise involving large muscle groups for

   a. 3 to 5 days per week, at 50–85% of max VO_2 for at least 10 minutes

   b. 4 to 6 days per week, at 70–90% of max VO_2 for at least 20 minutes

   c. 3 to 5 days per week, at 50–85% of max VO_2 for at least 15 minutes

   d. 4 to 6 days per week, at 60–90% of max VO_2 for at least 30 minutes

7. The major cause of coronary heart disease is
   a. stress
   b. atherosclerosis
   c. obesity
   d. diabetes
8. The elderly can benefit from exercise since it may
   a. reduce the muscular strength, bone mass and joint function lost with age
   b. prevent the reduction in aerobic capacity which occurs with age
   c. improve their intelligence
   d. a & b
9. The temporary cessation of a woman's monthly menstrual flow
   a. menarche
   b. menopause
   c. amenorrhea
   d. anorexia
10. Any behavior, or characteristic which may predispose one to disease
    a. bad habit
    b. risk factor
    c. epidemic
    d. genetic defect

Key Terms - Define the following terms:

1. Mortality
2. Healthy People 2000 objectives
3. Diabetes
4. Immunology
5. Menarche
6. Menopause
7. Amenorrhea
8. HDL-cholesterol
9. LDL-cholesterol
10. Risk Factor
11. Atherosclerosis
12. Thrombosis
13. RPE

Key Concepts - Review your lecture notes and the textbook. You should be able to answer the following questions:

♦ Differentiate between physical activity and exercise.

♦ Compare the health benefits obtained when moving from sedentary to moderately active to those of moving from moderately active to highly fit.

♦ Differentiate between health and fitness.

♦ List the known risk factors for coronary heart disease.

♦ Which of the coronary heart disease risk factors are linked to lifestyle?

♦ How much exercise is recommended to lower one's risk of disease?

♦ Compare the 1978 and 1990 recommendations for physical activity. Identify the differences and explain the apparent shift in our focus in regards to intensity, frequency, and duration.

♦ Differentiate between type I and type II diabetes.

♦ How is diabetes influenced by exercise?

♦ What are the current recommendations for pregnant women regarding exercise?

♦ Explain the relationship between hypertension and CHD.

♦ How does exercise influence one's risk profile for CHD?

♦ How are HDL and LDL different in regards to their influence on one's health?

♦ What can an individual do to decrease the number of risk factors they have for CHD?

Post Test

Multiple Choice

1. A medical condition, or habit associated with an increased risk of developing a specific health problem in the future
   a. bad habit
   b. risk factor
   c. genetic defect
   d. medical marker

2. The type of fitness associated with a lower mortality due to chronic diseases
   a. muscular strength
   b. muscular endurance
   c. flexibility
   d. cardiorespiratory

3. Physical activity and exercise are similar in that they both incorporate the
   a. expenditure of energy
   b. daily training regimens
   c. specific sport skills
   d. interval training

4. Sedentary lifestyles have been associated with all of the following except
   a. coronary heart disease
   b. colon cancer
   c. pancreatic cancer
   d. depression

5. The amount of activity one gets is a function of all of the following except
   a. intensity
   b. duration
   c. skill level
   d. frequency

6. The national health promotion and disease prevention objectives
   a. Wellness Guidelines 95
   b. Healthy People 2000
   c. Surgeon General's Report 95
   d. Wellness Guidelines 2000

7. Physical activity may help lower health costs by
   a. reducing accidents   b. preventing infectious disease
   c. reducing risk factors   d. preventing viral infections

8. A study by Lee et. al. showed lower all-cause mortality is reduced by exercise classified in the _____ range
   a. 1–2 METs   b. 3–4 METs
   c. 4–5 METs   d. > 6 METs

9. The majority of people in the United States die from one of these two diseases
   a. stroke, heart disease   b. cancer, stroke
   c. heart, pulmonary dysfunction d. cancer, heart disease

10. A slow progressive disease which involves a narrowing of the lumen of the arteries
    a. coronary heart disease   b. atherosclerosis
    c. coronary thrombosis   d. angina

11. Unstable angina or myocardial infarct result from
    a. asthma   b. emphysema
    c. thrombus formation   d. capillarization

12. Physical activity may lower cardiovascular mortality by all of the following except
    a. decreased stroke volume   b. increased electrical stability of myocardium
    c. increased contractility   d. decreased myocardial oxygen demand

13. The "big four" include all of the following except
    a. sedentary lifestyle   b. psychological stress
    c. smoking   d. elevated blood cholesterol

14. Treatment strategies for hypertension include all of the following except
    a. moderate exercise   b. medication
    c. decreased body weight   d. increased sodium intake

15. The majority of plasma lipids are packaged and transported in
    a. cholesterol esters   b. triglyceride esters
    c. lipoproteins   d. cholesterol-lipid esters

16. The formation of an atherosclerotic plaque involves all of the following except
    a. oxidation of LDL
    b. accumulation of cholesterol esters in macrophages
    c. reduction of LPL
    d. accumulation of cholesterol esters in smooth muscle cells

17. Particles which enter circulation devoid of cholesterol, and perform reverse cholesterol transport
    a. HDL   b. LDL_2
    c. LDL_3 d. VLDL

18. Stroke may result in loss of ability to express one's self, also known as
    a. hemiparesis   b. ataxia
    c. atrophy   d. aphasia

19. Blood-filled pouches which bulge from a weak spot in an artery wall
    a. thrombus   b. embolism
    c. aneurysm   d. aphasia

20. The type of cancer with the clearest inverse relationship with physical activity is
    a. liver   b. lung
    c. pancreatic   d. colon

21. Females experience _____, which is a cessation of menstruation due to hormonal changes
    a. menarche
    b. menopause
    c. luteal prolapse
    d. follicular failure

22. Obesity is known to be associated with a reduction in proteins which bind & transport
    a. zygotes
    b. follicles
    c. ovum
    d. estradiol

23. The ACSM classifies as apparently healthy, those persons without symptoms and ____ risk factors for coronary heart disease.
    a. no
    b. just one
    c. two
    d. both a & b

24. In 1994 the exercise for fitness paradigm was shifted to include exercise for
    a. health
    b. skill development
    c. pleasure
    d. beauty & weight loss

25. Subjective methods for prescribing exercise intensity might include which of the following?
    a. RPE scale
    b. talk test
    c. % VO_2 max
    d. METs

Answers - Chapter 14

Pretest

1. D
2. D
3. A
4. B
5. D
6. C
7. B
8. D
9. C
10. B

Post Test

1. B
2. D
3. A
4. C
5. C
6. B
7. C
8. D
9. D
10. B
11. C
12. A
13. B
14. D
15. C
16. C
17. A
18. D
19. C
20. D
21. B
22. D
23. D
24. A
25. A & B

CHAPTER 15
NUTRITION AND EXERCISE PERFORMANCE

Lecture Preparation: Multiple Choice

Instructions: After reading the chapter, read each question and the answer choices. Select the choice which BEST answers the question. Check your answers at the back of this chapter, and review any incorrectly answered questions in your textbook.

1.   The energy nutrients are
        a. carbohydrates   b. fats
        c. proteins   d. all of these answers

2.   Carbohydrate is stored in the body (as glycogen) in
        a. the blood   b. the muscles
        c. the liver   d. both b & c

3.   During anaerobic glycolysis, lactic acid results as an end product of glucose metabolism and is converted back to glucose by the liver in a process called
        a. the Krebs Cycle   b. the Glucose-Alanine Cycle
        c. the Cori Cycle   d. Beta Oxidation

4.   The structural difference between a saturated fatty acid and an unsaturated fatty acid is that
        a. an unsaturated fatty acid has at least one double bond
        b. a saturated fatty acid has at least one double bond
        c. an unsaturated fatty acid is unavailable to bind another hydrogen atom
        d. a saturated fatty acid has a double bond with a hydrogen atom

5.   Protein requirements for athletes are approximately
        a. 1.0–1.5 g. per kg. or 15% of their diet   b. 2.0–2.5 g. per kg. or 30% of their diet
        c. 5.0 g. per kg. or 30% of their diet   d. .5 g. per kg. or 20% of their diet

6.   The pregame meal should consist mainly of
        a. protein   b. carbohydrates
        c. fats   d. 50% protein and 50% carbohydrates

7.   The last meal prior to competition should be consumed
        a. within an hour before the event
        b. approximately 30 minutes prior to the event
        c. no later than 2 hours and thirty minutes prior to the event
        d. whenever the athlete desires, as the timing is not all that important

8.   The method of glycogen loading which results in the largest increase in glycogen storage is the procedure where
        a. a mixed diet is followed by 3 days of rest and high carbohydrate intake
        b. a period of exhaustive exercise is followed by 3 days of rest and high carbohydrate intake
        c. a period of low carbohydrate diet accompanied by exhaustive exercise is followed by 3 days of rest and high carbohydrate intake
        d. all of the above are equally effective

9.   Following an endurance activity, it is important for an athlete to eat a
a. meal high in carbohydrates and low in fat to replenish only the carbohydrates lost
b. well-balanced meal to replenish fat, carbohydrates, protein, vitamins and minerals lost
c. meal high in protein to replenish the amino acids lost
d. meal high in carbohydrates and fats to replenish kilocalories lost

10.   During prolonged exercise fluids can be ingested provided
I.   carbohydrate concentration does not exceed 4–8%
II.   water intake does not exceed 800 ml per hour
III. the water is lukewarm
IV.   the fluid replaced equals the fluid lost
a. I & II
b. I, II & III
c. II, III & IV
d. I, II, III & IV

11.   A nutrient which must be obtained directly through one's diet, may be classified as
a. nonessential   b. essential
c. micro   d. macro

12. Substances which donate electrons to help stabilize free radicals, are classified as
a. nonessential   b. essential
c. antiradicals   d. antioxidants

Key Terms - Define the following terms:

1.   Carbohydrate
2.   Lipid
3.   Protein
4.   Enzyme
5.   Fats
6.   Nutrients
7.   Nitrogen balance
8.   Vitamins
9.   Minerals
10. Antioxidants
11. Free radicals
12. Sports anemia
13. Anorexia Nervosa
14. Bulimia Nervosa

Key Concepts - Review your lecture notes and the textbook. You should be able to answer the following questions:

♦ Describe the basic structure of carbohydrates, fats, and protein.

♦ What criteria are used to classify a nutrient as essential or nonessential?

♦ Describe the role of vitamins and minerals in regards to exercise performance.

♦ What are the differences in dietary recommendations for athletes versus sedentary individuals?

♦ Describe the recommended pregame meal. What should be consumed, and when?

♦ Describe the recommended post event diet. What should be consumed, and when?

♦ What are the potential health related differences associated with consumption of water soluble and water insoluble fiber?

♦ Describe the current protein recommendations for sedentary people, endurance athletes, and strength athletes.

♦ What role do antioxidants play during exercise?

♦ Describe the basic methods utilized to load the muscles and liver with carbohydrates.

♦ What are the current recommendation regarding fluid ingestion before, during, and after competition?

Using the following information, outline the processes which occur for the glucose-alanine cycle and the Cori cycle.

The Cori cycle = 2 lactic acid molecules combined to produce glucose

The glucose-alanine cycle = conversion of alanine to glucose

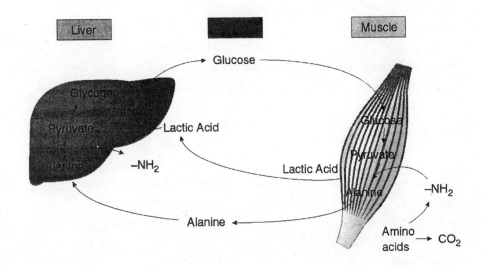

The glucose-alanine cycle involves _____

_____

_____

The Cori cycle involves _____

_____

_____

Post Test

Multiple Choice

1. Carbon, hydrogen, and oxygen make up the entire structure of
   - a. fats
   - b. protein
   - c. carbohydrates
   - d. both a & c

2. Monosaccharides include all of the following except
   - a. glucose
   - b. sucrose
   - c. fructose
   - d. galactose

3. The breakdown of glycogen into glucose is stimulated by
   - a. epinephrine
   - b. glucagon
   - c. insulin
   - d. both a & b

4. Glycogenesis and lipogenesis are stimulated by
   - a. epinephrine
   - b. glucagon
   - c. insulin
   - d. both a & b

5. Combining two molecules of lactic acid to form glucose occurs within the _____ cycle
   - a. Cori
   - b. glucose-alanine
   - c. lactate-glucose
   - d. none of these answers

6. The nondigestible portion of plant food is considered to be
   - a. carcinogenic
   - b. a waste
   - c. fiber
   - d. ketotic

7. The essential fatty acids are
   - a. alpha-linolenic
   - b. beta-linoleic
   - c. linoleic acid
   - d. linennic acid

8. A type of fatty acid which may decrease one's risk of heart disease is
   - a. palmitic acid
   - b. stearic acid
   - c. oleic acid
   - d. omega-3

9. A fatty acid containing one carbon to carbon double bond is classified as
   - a. a sterol
   - b. polyunsaturated
   - c. saturated
   - d. monounsaturated

10. Cholesterol is classified as a _____ type of lipid
    - a. sterol
    - b. polyunsaturated
    - c. saturated
    - d. monounsaturated

11. During long term endurance exercise proteins may contribute up to ____% of the energy required
    - a. 25
    - b. 15
    - c. 35
    - d. 50

12. The RDA for protein is ____ grams per kilogram of body weight per day
    - a. 0.08
    - b. 0.008
    - c. 0.80
    - d. 8.000

13. When an overabundance of amino acids are consumed, the extra amino acids are
    - a. converted into lean muscle mass
    - b. deaminated and converted into fat or glucose
    - c. stored in the liver
    - d. stored in the muscles

14. When an athlete is excreting more nitrogen than s/he is taking in, they are in
    a. negative nitrogen balance   b. positive nitrogen balance
    c. ketosis   d. nitrogen balance

15. During heavy weight lifting, the primary energy providing sources which help generate ATP are
    a. glucose & PC   b. glucose & fatty acids
    c. fatty acids & PC   d. leucine & isoleucine

16. Amino acids most readily available for energy metabolism include all of the following except
    a. leucine   b. isoleucine
    c. serine   d. valine

17. When a NH_2 radical combines with leucine, _____ is formed
    a. serine   b. alanine
    c. phenylalanine   d. glutamine

18. Supplementing one's diet with vitamins and minerals is generally believed to have ____ effect on athletic performance.
    a. a large positive   b. a large negative
    c. no evident   d. an ergogenic

19. Free radicals are molecules which are seeking
    a. electrons   b. protons
    c. neutrons   d. cations

20. Concerns with calcium consumption and athletes normally centers around
    a. their teeth   b. bone density
    c. amenorrhea   d. estradiol levels

21. Iron plays a role in athletic performance as a component of all of the following except
    a. hemoglobin   b. myoglobin
    c. CoA   d. cytochromes

22. The two **trace** minerals commonly lacking in athletes normal diets are
    a. calcium & phosphorous   b. chromium & zinc
    c. calcium & chromium   d. phosphorous & zinc

23. Athletes involved in sports emphasizing a lean appearance are at an increased risk for
    a. anemia   b. coronary heart disease
    c. eating disorders   d. chronic fatigue syndrome

24. The carbohydrate which is digested / absorbed most rapidly is
    a. glucose   b. fructose
    c. sucrose   d. lactose

25. The ingestion of large amounts (50–200 grams) of carbohydrates 30–60 minutes prior to exercise is now known to have what effect on performance for MOST athletes?
    a. it keeps glucose high for hours   b. no detrimental effect
    c. an insulin surge, then an energy burst   d. negative

Answers - Chapter 15

Pretest

1. D
2. D
3. C

4. A
5. A
6. B
7. C
8. C
9. B
10. A
11. B
12. D

Post Test

1. D
2. B
3. D
4. C
5. A
6. C
7. A & C
8. D
9. D
10. A
11. B
12. C
13. B
14. A
15. A
16. C
17. B
18. C
19. A
20. B
21. C
22. B
23. C
24. A
25. B

CHAPTER 16
EXERCISE, BODY COMPOSITION, AND WEIGHT CONTROL

Lecture Preparation: Multiple Choice

Instructions: After reading the chapter, read each question and the answer choices. Select the choice which BEST answers the question. Check your answers at the back of this chapter, and review any incorrectly answered questions in your textbook.

1. The somatotype classifications consist of a fatness component, muscle component and lean component termed

    a. mesomorph, ectomorph and endomorph, respectively

    b. endomorph, mesomorph and ectomorph, respectively

    c. ectomorph, mesomorph and endomorph, respectively

    d. ectomorph, endomorph and mesomorph, respectively

2. Body weight is gained when

    a. more energy is consumed than expended

    b. energy consumed equals the energy expended

    c. energy consumed is less than the energy expended

    d. none of the above can accurately predict weight gain

3. Underwater weighing and skinfold thickness can be measured to estimate one's

    a. body fat

    b. energy balance, positive or negative

    c. bone density

    d. all of the above

4. Athletes tend to have more

    a. mesomorph and ectomorph somatotype components then nonathletes

    b. endomorph and ectomorph somatotype components then nonathletes

    c. endomorph and mesomorph somatotype components then nonathletes

    d. typically have no significant somatotype different from that of nonathletes

5. The degree of obesity is dependent on

    a. the fat content of each fat cell and the number of fat cells

    b. the individual's body weight

    c. the location of the body fat

    d. age of onset

6. A wrestling coach could most accurately predict safe competitive weights by

    a. using anthropometric measures to predict each wrestler's minimal weight

    b. using the waist to hip ratio formula to predict each wrestler's minimal weight

    c. using height and weight charts to predict each wrestler's minimal weight

    d. all of the above are equally effective

7. As individuals age they tend to lose muscle mass, a process called

    a. middle age spread   b. sarcopenia

    c. freshman 15   d. creeping obesity

8.   Lean body mass is considered
        a. all mass which is non fat   b. muscle & bones only
        c. muscle, bones, & teeth only   d. all mass which contains nitrogen

Key Terms - Define the following terms:

1. Obesity

2. BMI

3. Adipocytes

4. Bioelectrical impedance

5. Body Density

6. Essential body fat

7. Lean body mass

8. Positive energy balance

9. Sarcopenia

Key Concepts - Review your lecture notes and the textbook. You should be able to answer the following questions:

+ Describe the three major categories for classifying body types using somatotyping procedures.

+ What is the importance of energy balance in maintaining one's weight?

+ Why is obesity viewed as having a negative effect upon one's overall health status?

+ Describe the basic differences between a lean and an obese individual's fat cells.

+ Why is underwater weighing considered the "gold standard" in measuring body fat?

+ Describe two other methods commonly used to determine percent body fat.

+ How does body fat influence athletic performance?

+ What is involved in "making weight"?

+ What recommendations does the ACSM make to decrease the incidence of wrestlers practicing harmful weight reduction techniques?

+ What did Tipton attempt to do for wrestlers?

Using the diagrams, indicate where each of the following skinfold sites would be taken. Draw a line to show the correct position and orientation of the fold.

1. Umbilical
2. Midaxillary
3. Subscapular

4. Tricep
5. Thigh
6. Chest

7. Abdominal
8. Suprailliac
9. Anterior axillary

10. Bicep
11. Calf

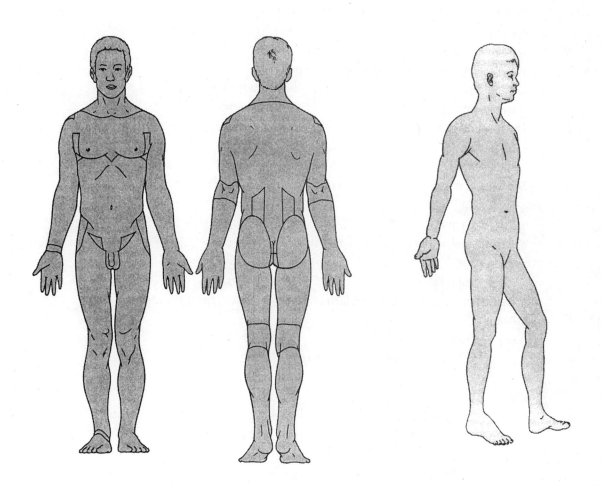

Post Test

Multiple Choice

1. The degree of obesity is dependent upon
   a. the number of fat cells
   b. the lipid content within the fat cells
   c. the location of fat cells
   d. both a & b

2. When an individual consumes fewer calories than they expend, they are in
   a. positive energy balance
   b. energy balance
   c. negative energy balance
   d. hypertrophy

3. The somatotype associated with soft, round portions of the body is
   a. ectomorph
   b. mesomorph
   c. endomorph
   d. somatomorph

4. The somatotype associated with an athletic, muscular appearance is
   a. ectomorph
   b. mesomorph
   c. endomorph
   d. somatomorph

5. The mass of the body divided by its volume gives us a measure of
   a. percent fat
   b. body density
   c. body mass index
   d. lean body mass

6. The traditional two compartment model divides the body into which of the following components?
   a. fat free body
   b. body fat
   c. subcutaneous fat
   d. essential fat

7. A method of measuring body fat which utilizes a low level electrical current is
   a. BMI
   b. skinfolds
   c. near infrared
   d. bioelectrical impedance

8. An individual is considered to be obese when their BMI is
   a. over 10
   b. over 25
   c. over 30
   d. over 20

9. During underwater weighing procedures one must take ____ into account.
   a. weight in the air
   b. weight in the water
   c. residual volume
   d. all of these variables

10. Equations which may be used to determine body density for a wide range of the population are considered
    a. rare
    b. generalized
    c. inappropriate
    d. specialized

11. When choosing an equation for measuring body fat via skinfolds, one must take into account
    a. gender
    b. athletic vs nonathletic
    c. in season vs off season
    d. both a & b

12. Obesity is related to all of the following except
    a. diabetes
    b. personality
    c. coronary heart disease
    d. hypertension

13. Authorities generally agree that one should maintain the weight attained between the ages of
    a. 12–16
    b. 16–19
    c. 19–22
    d. 25–30

14. The waist to hip circumference ratio is an indicator of
    a. central fat distribution
    b. peripheral fat distribution
    c. visceral fat content
    d. subcutaneous fat content

15. An increase in the number of fat cells
    a. hypertrophy
    b. hyperplasia
    c. adipocity
    d. adipoplasia

16. An increase in the size of fat cells
    a. hypertrophy
    b. hyperplasia
    c. adipocity
    d. adipoplasia

17. Evidence seems to support the following conclusion in regards to obesity
    a. treatment is easier than prevention
    b. prevention is easier than treatment
    c. treatment & prevention are equal
    d. treatment and prevention both fail

18. One's daily energy expenditure is equal to the sum of all of the following except
    a. dispersal energy
    b. basal energy expenditure
    c. energy for general activities
    d. energy cost of exercise

19. It requires _____ kcals to generate one additional pound of body fat.
    a. 2,000
    b. 2,500
    c. 3,000
    d. 3,500

20. It requires _____ kcals to generate one additional pound of lean body mass
    a. 2,000
    b. 2,500
    c. 3,000
    d. 3,500

21. Most athletes should not consume any fewer than _____ kcals per day.
    a. 1,000
    b. 1,500
    c. 1,800
    d. 3,500

22. While attempting to gain weight, one shouldn't exceed energy expenditure by more than ___ kcals per day.
    a. 100–200
    b. 300–400
    c. 500–1,000
    d. 1,000–1,500

23. Weight gaining attempts should be accompanied by
    a. extensive weight lifting
    b. extensive aerobic exercise
    c. interval training
    d. high protein shakes & raw egg whites

24. "Making weight" by dehydrating one's body leads to
    a. increased performance
    b. decreased upper body strength
    c. improved mental acuteness
    d. both a & c

25. Tipton concluded that wrestlers should
    a. obtain the lowest weight possible
    b. wrestle at a predetermined minimal weight
    c. ingest lipotropics to lose weight
    d. never reduce weight just to compete

Answers - Chapter 16

Pretest

1. B
2. A
3. A
4. A
5. A
6. A
7. B
8. A

Post Test

1. D
2. C
3. C
4. B
5. B
6. A & B
7. D
8. C
9. D
10. B
11. D
12. B
13. D
14. A
15. B
16. A
17. B
18. A
19. D
20. B
21. C
22. D
23. A
24. B
25. B

CHAPTER 17
EXERCISE AND THE ENDOCRINE SYSTEM

Lecture Preparation: Multiple Choice

Instructions: After reading the chapter, read each question and the answer choices. Select the choice which BEST answers the question. Check your answers at the back of this chapter, and review any incorrectly answered questions in your textbook.

1.   The _____ is often referred to as the master gland.
   a. hypothalamus   b. thalamus
   c. pituitary   d. thyroid

2.   Hormones are usually classified according to their
   a. size   b. activity level
   c. chemical composition   d. target tissue

3.   Releasing factors released by the _____, influence the secretion of many different hormones.
   a. hypothalamus   b. thalamus
   c. pituitary   d. thyroid

4.   The adrenal cortex is responsible for releasing
   a. mineralcorticoids   b. epinephrine
   c. glucocorticoids   d. both a & c

5.   The adrenal medulla is responsible for releasing
   a. mineralcorticoids   b. epinephrine
   c. glucocorticoids   d. both a & c

6.   The thyroid gland releases which of the following
   a. thyroxine   b. triiodothyronine
   c. cortisol   d. glucagon

7.   Thyroxine elevates the metabolism of many cells within the body by
   a. decreasing catecholamines   b. increasing receptor sites
   c. increasing blood sugar   d. increasing heart rate

8.   Hormones with a lipid based structure
   a. amino acid   b. cholesterol
   c. steroid   d. peptide

9.   The hormone which shows a decrease in blood concentration in response to exercise
   a. thyroxine   b. insulin
   c. cortisol   d. glucagon

10.   The pancreas plays a major role in regulating
   a. fat deposits   b. blood sugar
   c. overall metabolism   d. protein synthesis

11.   The primary androgenic hormone is
   a. thyroxine   b. estradiol
   c. cortisol   d. testosterone

12. Growth hormone levels during exercise
   a. rise sharply   b. rise slightly
   c. drop sharply   d. drop slightly

Key Terms - Define the following terms:

1. Hormone

2. Receptor site

3. Second messenger

4. Negative feedback

5. Trophic hormone

6. Hypothalamus

7. Adenohypophysis

8. Neurohypophysis

9. Catecholamine

10. Mineral corticoids

11. Glucocorticoids

12. Steroid hormones

13. Cyclic AMP

Key Concepts - Review your lecture notes and the textbook. You should be able to answer the following questions:

♦ Describe the manner in which hormones interact with target cells.

♦ How do second messengers play a role in hormone induced reactions?

♦ List the endocrine glands and the hormones which they secrete.

♦ Describe the basic physiological response of the body to the presence of increased levels of each hormone listed in the above response.

♦ Describe the changes experienced due to exercise for each hormone listed above.

♦ Describe the influence of training on each specific hormone's level.

Using the words from the word bank, label the endocrine glands on the drawing. Below each gland, list the hormones which are secreted by the gland.

Word Bank

Thyroid	Pituitary	Hypothalamus	Adrenal cortex	Adrenal medulla
Pancreas	Testes	Ovaries	Parathyroid	Thymus
Thyroxine	Epinephrine	Norepinephrine	Glucagon	Insulin
Estrogen	Testosterone	Calcatonin	Cortisol	Growth hormone
ACTH	ADH	Aldosterone	Releasing factors	

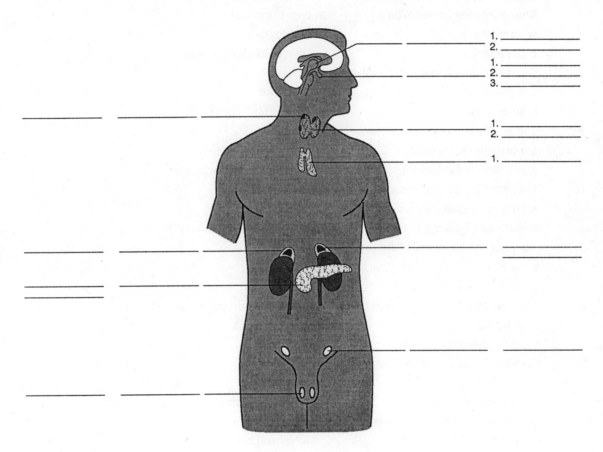

1. _____
2. _____

1. _____
2. _____
3. _____

_____

1. _____
2. _____

1. _____

_____   _____

_____

_____

_____

Post Test

Multiple Choice

1. A discrete chemical substance secreted into the body fluids by an endocrine gland
   a. cAMP
   b. second messenger
   c. endocrine messenger
   d. hormone

2. The endocrine system may have all of the following effects on target tissues except
   a. activates enzyme systems
   b. alters cell membrane permeability
   c. stimulates protein synthesis
   d. initiates NEW reactions

3. Most hormones interact with _____ at their target tissue.
   a. receptor site
   b. enzymes
   c. lipoproteins
   d. special phospholipids

4. One of the most important second messengers is
   a. thyroxine
   b. cAMP
   c. aldosterone
   d. cortisol

5. The secretion of hormones is precisely regulated via
   a. a feed forward response
   b. negative feedback
   c. cell mediated interruption
   d. the hormones available

6. The secretion of many hormones is under the influence of the
   a. hormone regulating peptides
   b. nervous system
   c. hormone regulating factors
   d. none of these answers

7. The pituitary releases all of the following except
   a. cortisol
   b. ADH
   c. GH
   d. TSH

8. The sympathetic nervous system releases ____ from its postganglionic fibers.
   a. catecholamines
   b. epinephrine
   c. norepinephrine
   d. dopamine

9. Catecholamines are released from the
   a. thyroid gland
   b. pancreas
   c. adrenal cortex
   d. adrenal medulla

10. Electrolyte metabolism is regulated in part by _____ hormones.
    a. glucocorticoid
    b. mineral corticoid
    c. steroid
    d. liver

11. All of the following are effects of cortisol except
    a. blunted insulin action
    b. increased gluconeogenesis
    c. anti-inflammatory response
    d. increased lipogenesis

12. The tight regulation of blood sugar is performed by
    a. insulin & somatostatin
    b. glucagon & somatostatin
    c. glucagon & insulin
    d. insulin & growth hormone

13. The hormones responsible for a general increase in metabolism are
    a. insulin & somatostatin
    b. thyroxin & triiodothyronine
    c. thyroxin & insulin
    d. thyroxin & somatostatin

14. Calcium levels are regulated by
   a. insulin & glucagon
   b. thyroxin & triiodothyronine
   c. parathyroid hormone & calcitonin
   d. calcitonin & somatostatin

15. Red blood cell production is increased in the presence of
   a. insulin
   b. erythropoietin
   c. erythrocytosis
   d. somatostatin

16. The ____ are a class of substances which stimulate the growth of muscle and cartilage.
   a. somatomedins
   b. somatostatin
   c. prostaglandins
   d. none of these answers

17. Changes in the level of specific hormones circulating during exercise is caused by
   a. altered secretion
   b. altered metabolic turnover rates
   c. hemoconcentration
   d. all of these answers

18. Training influences the release of growth hormone in response to exercise in the following way
   a. it decreases
   b. it increases
   c. there is no training effect
   d. it is a biphasic response

19. Hormones such as thyroxin and cortisol are influenced by which of the following exercise factors?
   a. intensity
   b. duration
   c. fitness level
   d. all of these answers

20. The release of aldosterone and renin is caused by all of the following except
   a. sodium loss
   b. decreased plasma volume
   c. decreased plasma osmolarity
   d. increased sympathetic activity

21. Training influences blood catecholamine levels by
   a. decreasing them at rest
   b. blunting their rise during submaximal exercise
   c. increasing them at rest
   d. increasing them during submaximal exercise

22. The levels of circulating insulin _____.
   a. increase significantly with exercise
   b. decrease during exercise
   c. are not influenced by exercise
   d. increase slightly during exercise

23. The substances classified as _____ promote vasodilation
   a. endorphins
   b. somatomedins
   c. prostaglandins
   d. ergogenic

24. Most hormones are _____ in circulating levels during exercise
   a. increased
   b. decreased
   c. unaltered
   d. biphasic

25. Many hormones show an increased blood concentration during exercise. Exception(s) to this is/are
   a. insulin
   b. endorphins
   c. catecholamines
   d. both a & b

Answers - Chapter 17

Pretest

1. C
2. C
3. A

4. D
5. B
6. A & B
7. B
8. C
9. B
10. B
11. D
12. B

Post Test

1. D
2. D
3. A
4. B
5. B
6. B
7. A
8. C
9. D
10. B
11. D
12. C
13. B
14. C
15. B
16. A
17. D
18. A
19. D
20. C
21. B
22. B
23. C
24. A
25. D

CHAPTER 18
DRUGS AND ERGOGENIC AIDS

Lecture Preparation:

Instructions: After reading the chapter, read each question and the answer choices. Select the choice which BEST answers the question. Check your answers at the back of this chapter, and review any incorrectly answered questions in your textbook.

For each potential ergogenic aid listed below, match it with the theoretical mechanism as described below (place this letter in the first blank). In the second blank place a + (plus) if research shows it works under any conditions, place a – (minus) in the space if it has not been shown to work.

1.____ Anabolic androgenic steroids ____

2.____ Creatine supplements ____

3.____ L-Carnitine ____

4.____ Beta$_2$-agonists ____

5.____ Bicarbonate loading ____

6.____ Caffeine ____

7.____ Clenbutarol ____

8.____ Ephedrine ____

9.____ DHEA (**DeHydroEpiAndrosterone**) ____

10.____ Erythropoietin ____

11.____ Ginseng ____

12.____ BCAA ____

A. A substance which serves to help buffer intracellular acidity.

B. A substance which serves as a reservoir for phosphates, aids in energy production.

C. A substance which may help stimulate production of new RBCs.

D. Substances which increase activity of receptor sites predominantly found in skeletal muscles.

E. A stimulant, not commonly found in foods, which increases alertness.

F. A stimulant, commonly found in foods, which increases the mobilization of free fatty acids.

G. A hormone which promotes cell division & growth, claimed to reduce aging process.

H. Herbal product which is often claimed to be an anti-aging phytochemical.

I. A protein substance which helps transport fatty acids across the mitochondrial membrane.

J. A substance which is often used as a steroid replacement.

K. A hormone-based substance which promotes protein synthesis, enables one to recover quickly from exercise.

L. Claimed to slow the entry of tryptophan into the brain, preventing increases in serotonin, thus delaying fatigue.

Key Terms - Define the following terms:

1. Ergogenic aid

2. Double blind study

3. Placebo effect

4. Ergolytic effect

Ergogenic Substances - for each substance listed, describe the theoretical basis for its use as an ergogenic aid, then discuss whether the research verifies any proposed ergogenic properties.

- ♦ Anabolic-androgenic steroids
- ♦ Amphetamines
- ♦ Beta$_2$-agonists
- ♦ Bicarbonate loading
- ♦ Branch-chain amino acids
- ♦ Carnitine
- ♦ Caffeine
- ♦ Creatine
- ♦ Ephedrine
- ♦ Erythropoietin
- ♦ Ginseng
- ♦ Sympathomimetic amines

Key Concepts - Review your lecture notes and the textbook. You should be able to answer the following questions:

- ♦ Describe some of the problems associated with our attempts to assess current literature regarding ergogenic aids. How can we interpret the data? How do we know what is accurate, etc.?

- ♦ List 3 potential factors creating fatigue (physiological factors only)

- ♦ What is meant by doping?

- ♦ What are the criteria used to determine whether a substance is ergogenic?

- ♦ List the various categories into which ergogenic aids may be grouped.

- ♦ Describe some of the problems encountered by scientists examining the ergogenic effect of various substances.

- ♦ How can a substance be ergolytic?

- ♦ How can an athlete determine if a particular substance will help improve their performance?

Post Test

Multiple Choice

1. Ergogenic effects may be achieved by all of the following except
   a. delay the onset of fatigue
   b. supply fuel
   c. decrease nervous system activity
   d. act directly on muscle

2. An inert substance which has identical physical characteristics to a real drug is considered
   a. placebo
   b. double blind
   c. ergogenic
   d. ergolytic

3. Carbohydrate loading is often associated with
   a. increased fat mass
   b. increased water retention
   c. increased protein synthesis
   d. decreased protein synthesis

4. Supplementing with vitamins will generally _____ one's performance.
   a. increase
   b. decrease
   c. not influence
   d. contribute to

5. Anabolic-androgenic steroids have ___ & ___ properties.
   a. growth & catabolic
   b. growth & masculinizing
   c. growth & feminizing
   d. none of these answers

6. Side effects from steroids include all of the following except
   a. acne
   b. liver ailments
   c. decreased blood lipids
   d. decreased sperm production

7. The effects of _____ are similar to those achieved via anabolic steroids.
   a. caffeine
   b. chromium
   c. growth hormone
   d. carnitine

8. Amphetamines are drugs which
   a. increase sympathetic nervous system activity
   b. increase parasympathetic system activity
   c. improve endurance performance
   d. reduce anxiety

9. Ingesting large quantities of bicarbonate has been shown to
   a. decrease resting heart rate
   b. increase stroke volume
   c. cause vasodilation
   d. buffer lactic acid

10. Caffeine may be ergogenic via its
    a. decreasing protein synthesis
    b. increasing protein synthesis
    c. directly increasing beta oxidation
    d. increasing mobilization of FFA

11. For blood doping to elicit an ergogenic effect, at least_____ ml of blood must be reinfused.
    a. 200–300
    b. 400–500
    c. 600–800
    d. 800–1,200

12. All of the following are risks associated with blood doping except
    a. thrombosis
    b. viral infection
    c. air embolism
    d. anemia

13. Breathing pure oxygen prior to a running event will _____ performance
    a. increase
    b. decrease
    c. not influence
    d. modify

14. Clenbutarol is classified as a
    a. narcotic
    b. $beta_2$-agonist
    c. depressant
    d. steroid

15. The substance which proposes to increase fat use as a fuel by helping transport FA across the mitochondrial membrane is
    a. carnitine
    b. creatine
    c. choline
    d. ephedrine

16. The substance which many claim will prevent fatigue by increasing the quantity of neurotransmitter available for muscle contraction is
    a. carnitine
    b. choline
    c. creatine
    d. chromium

17. Branch-chain amino acids are proposed as ergogenic in that they may
    a. delay fatigue   b. increase muscle size
    c. increase PC levels   d. delay muscle soreness
18. Phosphate loading is potentially ergogenic in that it may help
    a. increase muscle size   b. serve as a buffer
    c. increase PC levels   d. delay muscle soreness
19. Vitamins which may play a role as antioxidants include all of the following except
    a. beta carotene   b. vitamin C
    c. vitamin E   d. vitamin D
20. Why do weight lifters often ingest large quantities of amino acids?
    a. they can't ingest adequate amounts through their diet
    b. to increase muscle mass
    c. these proteins are superior to those found in food
    d. to prevent fatigue

Answers - Chapter 18

Pretest

1. k,+
2. b,+
3. i,-
4. d,+
5. a,+
6. f,+
7. j,+
8. e+1
9. g,-
10. c,+
11. h,-
12. l,-

Post Test

1. C
2. A
3. B
4. C
5. B
6. C
7. C
8. A
9. D
10. D
11. D
12. D
13. C
14. B
15. A
16. B
17. A
18. B
19. D
20. B

CHAPTER 19
TEMPERATURE REGULATION: EXERCISE IN HEAT AND COLD

Lecture Preparation: Multiple Choice

Instructions: After reading the chapter, read each question and the answer choices. Select the choice which BEST answers the question. Check your answers at the back of this chapter, and review any incorrectly answered questions in your textbook.

1.   The two major thermal receptors in the body are found

      a. in the hypothalamus and in skeletal muscles

      b. in the hypothalamus and the skin

      c. in the skin and in skeletal muscles

      d. along the lumen of arterial blood vessels and in skeletal muscles

2.   In the body heat is transferred

      a. down the temperature gradient from the muscle, to the core, to the skin

      b. by radiation and convection from the skin to the environment depending on the temperature gradient between the skin and the air

      c. by evaporation from the skin to the environment dependent on the difference in vapor pressure between the skin and the environment

      d. all of the above

3.   Peripheral vasoconstriction

    I.   shunts blood from the skin to the core

    II.   is a physiological response to heat exposure

    III. shunts blood from the core to the skin

    IV. is a physiological response to cold exposure

        a. I & II

        b. I & IV

        c. II & III

        d. III & IV

4.   Subcutaneous fat serves as the most important natural insulator in humans because

      a. it covers vital organs

      b. it is metabolized easily at rest to produce heat

      c. it has low conductivity due to low vascularization

      d. all of the above

5.   Heat illnesses in athletics can be significantly reduced through

      a. heat acclimatization

      b. proper clothing

      c. fluid and electrolyte replacement

      d. all of the above

6. If a person exercising is burning 10 kcals per minute, they are producing
   a. enough heat to raise a kilogram of water 10 degrees Centigrade
   b. enough heat to raise their body temperature 10 degrees Centigrade
   c. both a & b
   d. neither a or b

7. Physiological changes occurring within an individual in order to adjust to changes in the natural environment are classified under the term
   a. acclimation   b. climadaption
   c. acclimatization   d. none of the above

8. Acute adjustments that take place in the body in response to stressful changes in climate are classified under the term
   a. acclimation   b. climadaption
   c. acclimatization   d. none of the above

9. Reduced sweating, hot skin, tachycardia, and seizures are signs of
   a. heat stroke a life threatening heat illness
   b. heat exhaustion a dangerous heat illness
   c. heat cramping a common and somewhat mild heat illness
   d. heat syncope a dangerous heat illness.

10. The mechanisms used by the body to give off heat include which of the following?
    a. conduction   b. convection
    c. radiation   d. evaporation

11. Windchill is determined by factoring in both
    a. wind & rain   b. wind and ice
    c. wind & air temperature   d. wind & water temperature

12. When an individual's body becomes extremely cold, they are in danger of experiencing
    a. hyperthermia   b. windchill
    c. hypothermia   d. dehydration

Key Terms - Define the following terms:

1. Heat balance
2. Evaporation
3. Conduction
4. Convection
5. Radiation
6. Thermal receptors
7. Dehydration
8. Acclimation
9. Hypothermia
10. Hyperthermia
11. Windchill
12. Heat syncope
13. Heat cramps
14. Heat stroke
15. Heat exhaustion

Key Concepts - Review your lecture notes and the textbook. You should be able to answer the following questions:

♦ How does the body readjust its physiological processes to maintain thermal homeostasis?

♦ What mechanisms are utilized to sense temperature changes throughout the body?

♦ What is the role of the hypothalamus in regulating body temperature?

♦ What mechanisms are utilized to release heat from the body to the environment?

♦ Describe the signs and symptoms of the various heat related illnesses.

♦ What physiological adjustments are made as one acclimates to a warmer or a colder environment?

♦ What factors need to be considered when scheduling an athletic event in either a warm or a cold environment?

♦ How does fuel utilization change as a result of temperature changes?

♦ How do children and adults differ in their overall response to warm or cold environments?

♦ How do changes in environmental and core temperatures alter the oxygen cost of an activity?

♦ How might one avoid heat related illnesses?

♦ How might cold related problems be avoided?

♦ Describe how one's sweat composition changes as a result of acclimating to a hot environment.

♦ Describe the best way to dress for exercise in a cold environment.

♦ How is one's sweating rate and pattern altered by heat acclimation?

♦ How does the sweat response of females compare to that of males?

Examine the diagram carefully, then indicate in the boxes the mechanism by which heat is being transferred.

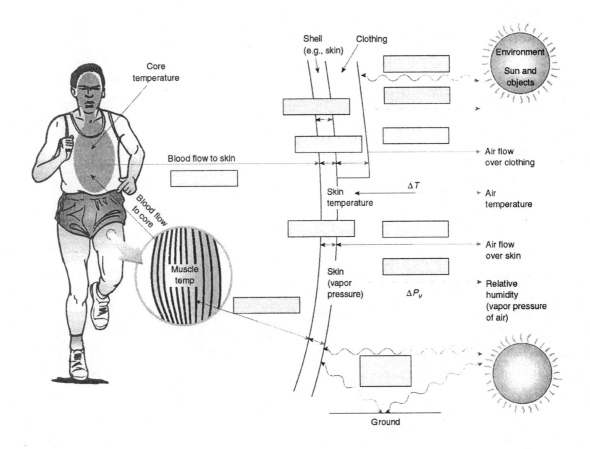

Fill in the boxes using the terms, evaporation, conduction, convection, and radiation.

Post Test

Fill in the blank

1. Differences in the physiological responses of males versus females to heat and cold are probably best explained by differences in _____.

2. The transfer of heat through electromagnetic waves is referred to as _____.

3. Central thermal receptors are located in the _____.

4. Heat loss through the head, during exercise, may be significant, or up to _____ % of total heat loss.

5. The energy cost of submaximal work is _____ due to shivering while exercising.

6. Wind _____ and temperature are used to determine the windchill.

7. Older individuals have a _____ heat tolerance than younger people.

8. The heat disorder characterized by spasms or twitching in the arms or legs, and possibly the abdomen is called _____.

9. The heat disorder characterized by "cotton mouth", weakness, loss of coordination, elevated core and skin temperature, and very concentrated urine is _____.

10. The heat disorder characterized by vomiting, diarrhea, elevated core and skin temperature, seizures, and coma is _____.

Multiple Choice

1. Body heat is lost through all of the following except
   a. evaporation   b. conduction
   c. convection   d. acclimation

2. Transfer of heat from one place to another by the movement of a heated substance
   a. evaporation   b. conduction
   c. convection   d. acclimation

3. The transfer of heat between two objects which are in direct contact with one another
   a. evaporation   b. conduction
   c. convection   d. radiation

4. The type of sweat glands which are most numerous & secrete a watery fluid
   a. apocrine   b. eccrine
   c. endocrine   d. none of these answers

5. The formation and secretion of sweat is known as
   a. hidropoesis   b. dehydration
   c. acclimation   d. poresis

6. Sweating cools the body via
   a. radiation   b. conduction
   c. convection   d. evaporation

7. Heat is carried from the muscles & core of the body to the surface via the blood. This process is an example of heat loss via
   a. evaporation   b. conduction
   c. convection   d. radiation

8. The thermal regulatory center is located in the
   a. hypothalamus
   b. pituitary
   c. brain stem
   d. medulla oblongata

9. Tissues which are sensitive to changes in temperature are regarded as
   a. thermal regulatory centers
   b. thermal effectors
   c. thermal receptors
   d. thermal organs

10. Each of the following is a thermal effector except
    a. sweat glands
    b. skeletal muscles
    b. thyroid gland
    d. liver

11. Higher heart rates while exercising at the same intensity in hot environments is due to
    a. increased cardiac output
    b. decreased stroke volume
    c. increased end diastolic volume
    d. decreased afterload

12. Which of the following is the most serious heat related problem?
    a. heat syncope
    b. heat cramps
    c. heat stroke
    d. heat exhaustion

13. Persons particularly prone to heat illness include which of the following?
    a. obese
    b. children
    c. those with prior heat illness
    d. unfit individuals

14. Training in the heat will alter sweating patterns such that sweating will begin _____ (in comparison to preacclimatization)
    a. at lower core temperatures
    b. at higher core temperatures
    c. at lower ambient temperatures
    d. at higher ambient temperatures

15. Sweat composition is altered after training in the heat such that it contains
    a. more potassium
    b. less sodium
    c. more iron
    d. less water

16. Fluids for rehydration or sports drinks should be
    a. cool
    b. palatable
    c. hypotonic
    d. readily available

17. Each of the following responses occurs while exposed to the cold except
    a. shivering
    b. peripheral vasoconstriction
    c. decreased catecholamines
    d. increased nonshivering thermogenesis

18. When core temperature is lowered an individual will experience a(n)
    a. decreased aerobic capacity
    b. increased aerobic capacity
    c. increased total work capacity
    d. no change in aerobic work capacity

19. Muscle glycogen is used at a higher rate in cold environments due to
    a. reduced FFA release from adipocytes
    b. reduced PC levels
    c. reduced ATP levels
    d. reduced intramuscular triglyceride stores

20. The irritation of the throat while exercising in the cold is due to the
    a. lungs freezing
    b. drying of the mucosal tissue
    c. slowed action of cilia
    d. accumulation of moisture in the throat

21.   Those individuals more prone to shiver and experience discomfort in the cold include
a. lean individuals   b. obese individuals
c. children   d. both a & c

22.   Chronic physiological changes which allow an individual to adjust to changes in their natural environment
a. acclimation   b. acclimatization
c. assimilation   d. accommodation

23.   Physiological changes due to acute exposure to environmental changes
a. acclimation   b. acclimatization
c. assimilation   d. accommodation

24.   The cooling convective power of the environment is taken into account by the _____ index
a. frostbite   b. shivering
c. windchill   d. wet bulb

25.   A standardized insulating unit is the _____. It represents the amount of insulating material required to keep a person comfortable.
a. windchill index   b. clo
c. clothing index   d. shivering index

Answers - Chapter 19

Pretest

1. B
2. D
3. B
4. C
5. D
6. A
7. C
8. A
9. A
10. A, B, C, D
11. C
12. C

Post Test

Fill in the blank

1. body composition
2. radiation
3. hypothalamus
4. 30%
5. elevated

6. velocity

7. lower

8. heat cramps

9. heat exhaustion

10. heat stroke

Multiple choice

1. D

2. C

3. B

4. B

5. A

6. D

7. C

8. A

9. B

10. D

11. B

12. C

13. A, B, C, D

14. A

15. B

16. A, B, C, D

17. C

18. A

19. A

20. B

21. D

22. B

23. A

24. C

25. B

CHAPTER 20
PERFORMANCE UNDERWATER, AT HIGH ALTITUDE, AND DURING AND AFTER MICROGRAVITY

Lecture Preparation: Multiple Choice

Instructions: After reading the chapter, read each question and the answer choices. Select the choice which BEST answers the question. Check your answers at the back of this chapter, and review any incorrectly answered questions in your textbook.

1. Diffusion is
    a. the random movement of particles caused by the kinetic energy of the particle
    b. the movement of particles from an area of higher concentration to lower
    c. the most important means by which particles move into and out of the cell
    d. all of the above

2. The law that states when the temperature of a given volume of gas is increased, the volume increases is
    a. Boyle's Law
    b. Charles's Law
    c. Dalton's Law
    d. Henry's Law

3. The law that deals with the inverse relationship between the pressure of a gas and the volume of gas is
    a. Boyle's Law
    b. Charles's Law
    c. Dalton's Law
    d. Henry's Law

4. The law that state that partial pressures of gases in a mixture remain constant and act independently of each other is
    a. Boyle's Law
    b. Charles's Law
    c. Dalton's Law
    d. Henry's Law

5. The law that refers to the direct relationship between the partial pressure of a gas and the amount of gas a fluid will absorb is
    a. Boyle's Law
    b. Charles's Law
    c. Dalton's Law
    d. Henry's Law

6. When first arriving at a higher altitude, a person's pH will usually rise due to
    a. an increased red blood cell count
    b. increased oxidative enzymes and mitochondrial density
    c. increased muscle and tissue capillarization
    d. hyperventilation

7. To increase the oxygen content of the arterial blood the body at altitude or under conditions where there is a lower PO_2

   a. increases the plasma volume

   b. produces more red blood cells

   c. decreases pulmonary ventilation

   d. eliminates the excretion of bicarbonate

8. At altitudes over 5000 feet, endurance performance is decreased due to

   a. hypoxia resulting from lower PO_2

   b. hypoventilation

   c. decreased pH

   d. all of the above

9. Upon a diver's rapid ascent to regions of lower pressure, a dangerous condition in which nitrogen gas emboli can cause a circulatory blockage is called

   a. nitrogen narcosis

   b. nitrogen poisoning

   c. the bends

   d. the shakes

10. Oxygen poisoning results from

   a. application of Henry's Law in reference to oxygen being forced into the plasma when using 100% oxygen during underwater diving

   b. the inability for the red blood cell to transport CO_2 back to the alveoli

   c. the inability for the red blood cells to adequately off-load O_2 at the tissues

   d. all of the above

Key Terms - Define the following terms:

1. Hyperbaric

2. Barometric pressure

3. Microgravity

4. Air embolus

5. Spontaneous pneumothorax

6. The bends

7. Nitrogen narcosis

8. Oxygen poisoning

9. Boyle's Law

10. Charles's Law

11. Dalton's Law

12. Henry's Law

13. Penquin suit

14. Microgravity

Key Concepts - Review your lecture notes and the textbook. You should be able to answer the following questions:

- How do temperature and pressure interact to influence the volume of a gas?

- Describe the conditions which will cause one to get the bends.

- Explain how oxygen can actually become detrimental to one's health in hyperbaric environments.

- What situations could potentially lead to spontaneous pneumothorax?

- What conditions predispose one to experience nitrogen narcosis?

- How does water differ from air in relationship to pressure?

- How does microgravity influence physiological processes?

- How does altitude alter ventilation and oxygen consumption?

- What influence does altitude have on performance?

- Does altitude training improve endurance performance? Explain the rationale for your answer.

Examine each series of pictures. Using your text, indicate which of the following conditions is occuring and then which gas law best explains the event.

<u>Conditions</u>

The bends

Spontaneous pneumothorax

Formation of an emboli

<u>Gas Laws</u>

Boyle's Law

Charles's Law

Henry's Law

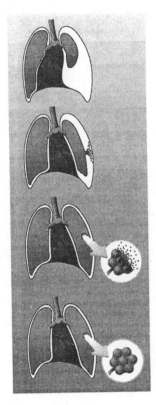

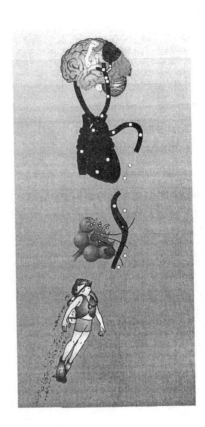

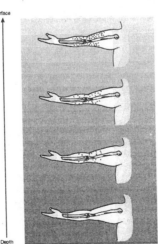

Post Test

Fill in the blank

1. Lack of adequate oxygen results in _____.

2. The oxygen cost of swimming underwater is _____ than on the surface.

3. As one descends underwater, the pressure on their body _____.

4. Because the body is mainly water, it is _____ compressible.

5. If air bubbles form in the blood, they are called _____.

6. The lowered PO_2 at altitude will elicit a(n)_____ in the ventilatory response.

7. Cardiac output increases at altitude due to an increase in _____.

8. Altitude may increase pulmonary blood pressure. This may result in altitude sickness or _____.

9. Moderate altitude training should be mixed periodically with _____ altitude training.

10. Muscle cross-sectional area _____ in response to long term microgravity exposure.

Multiple choice

1. When the pressure on a given volume of gas is doubled, the volume
   a. increases by one half
   b. is reduced by one half
   c. increases in an unknown way
   d. is reduced by one tenth

2. The relationship between the volume and pressure of a gas is explained by
   a. Boyle's Law
   b. Henry's Law
   c. Dalton's Law
   d. Charles's Law

3. Heating a gas will cause it to
   a. explode
   b. expand
   c. implode
   d. compress

4. The relationship between temperature and the volume of a gas is explained by
   a. Boyle's Law
   b. Henry's Law
   c. Dalton's Law
   d. Charles's Law

5. Water is
   a. virtually non-compressible
   b. incomprehensible
   c. very compressible
   d. always the same density

6. As one descends under water, one additional atmosphere of pressure occurs every ____ feet of depth.
   a. 14
   b. 28
   c. 33
   d. 64

7. The relationship between partial pressures of gases within a mixture are explained by
   a. Boyle's Law
   b. Henry's Law
   c. Dalton's Law
   d. Charles's Law

8. As one descends underwater and the pressure increases, the amount of gases absorbed by the blood
   a. remains unchanged
   b. increases
   c. dissociates
   d. decreases

9. Partial pressure of a given volume of gas is equal to the product of
   a. total pressure & fractional concentration
   b. atmospheric pressure & fractional concentration
   c. total pressure & volume
   d. volume & fractional concentration

10. Increased altitude influences air in which of the following ways?
    a. decreases the weight of air
    b. increases the weight of air
    c. increases fractional concentration
    d. decreases fractional concentration

11. Quickly releasing or removing the pressure from a liquid with gases dissolved in it will result in
    a. oxygen poisoning
    b. nitrogen narcosis
    c. bubbles forming
    d. spontaneous pneumothorax

12. One of the most important things to remember when scuba diving is to
    a. recall where the boat is located
    b. exhale while descending
    c. inhale while ascending
    d. exhale while ascending

13. An accumulation of air in the pleural cavity occurs with
    a. oxygen poisoning
    b. nitrogen narcosis
    c. pulmonary embolism
    d. spontaneous pneumothorax

14. Nitrogen narcosis occurs due to the increased nitrogen in solution within the body, influencing the
    a. CNS
    b. skeletal muscles
    c. respiratory system
    d. heart

15. A condition called the bends occurs when divers
    a. run out of oxygen
    b. ascend too quickly
    c. descend too quickly
    d. fail to mix nitrogen into their tank

16. Symptoms of the bends include all of the following except
    a. pain in legs & arms
    b. paralysis
    c. bubbles escaping from the lungs
    d. unconsciousness

17. Successful treatment for the bends involves
    a. inserting a hypodermic needle into the pleural cavity
    b. returning to their diving depth and ascending more quickly
    c. entering a compression chamber, then decompressing slowly
    d. breathing pure oxygen

18. The actual physiological problem associated with oxygen poisoning is
    a. there is too much oxygen loaded onto the hemoglobin & oxygen becomes toxic
    b. excess oxygen diffuses into tissues causing one to feel intoxicated
    c. oxygen diffuses into the brain and creates dizziness
    d. dissolved oxygen is utilized, oxygen remains on the hemoglobin preventing adequate CO_2 removal

19. At altitude the oxygen in the air
    a. remains the same percentage
    b. decreases in percentage
    c. increases in percentage
    d. is better able to bind to hemoglobin

20. The major problems noted with long term microgravity include all of the following except
    a. bone demineralization
    b. muscle atrophy
    c. connective tissue loss
    d. cardiovascular deconditioning

21. Astronauts wear a penquin suit in an effort to
    a. keep oxygen at proper levels
    b. maintain resistive stress on muscles
    c. keep from floating away
    d. maintain waste elimination
22. The following occur due to altitude acclimatization except
    a. increased number of RBCs
    b. elimination of bicarbonate in the urine
    c. increased capillarization
    d. retention of bicarbonate by the kidneys
23. Most studies reveal that when elite athletes train at altitude, their sea level performance will
    a. increase
    b. decrease
    c. not improve
    d. it remains controversial
24. Altitude training guidelines recommend that important athletic contests be performed about_____ days after returning to sea level.
    a. 0–1
    b. 2–5
    c. 6–10
    d. 14
25. The altitude training guidelines recommend that the bulk of training time should be spent
    a. lifting weights
    b. at very high altitude
    c. at moderate altitude
    d. performing plyometrics

Answers - Chapter 20

Pretest

1. B
2. B
3. A
4. C
5. D
6. D
7. B
8. A
9. C
10. B

Post Test

Fill in the blank

1. hypoxia
2. greater
3. increases
4. not
5. emboli
6. increase
7. heart rate
8. pulmonary edema

9. high

10. decreases

Multiple choice

1. B
2. A
3. B
4. D
5. A
6. C
7. C
8. B
9. A
10. A
11. C
12. D
13. D
14. A
15. B
16. C
17. C
18. D
19. A
20. C
21. B
22. D
23. C
24. D
25. C